FINDING INNER

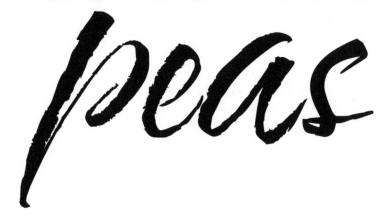

peas

My Sometimes-Hilarious Story of Infertility,
High-Risk Pregnancy, and Finding Out
That I Control Absolutely Nothing.

ERIN SALEM

BALBOA.
PRESS
A DIVISION OF HAY HOUSE

Balboa Press books may be ordered through booksellers or by contacting:

Balboa Press
A Division of Hay House
1663 Liberty Drive
Bloomington, IN 47403
www.balboapress.com
1 (877) 407-4847

Because of the dynamic nature of the Internet, any web addresses or links contained in this book may have changed since publication and may no longer be valid. The views expressed in this work are solely those of the author and do not necessarily reflect the views of the publisher, and the publisher hereby disclaims any responsibility for them.

The author of this book does not dispense medical advice or prescribe the use of any technique as a form of treatment for physical, emotional, or medical problems without the advice of a physician, either directly or indirectly. The intent of the author is only to offer information of a general nature to help you in your quest for emotional and spiritual well-being. In the event you use any of the information in this book for yourself, which is your constitutional right, the author and the publisher assume no responsibility for your actions.

Any people depicted in stock imagery provided by Getty Images are models, and such images are being used for illustrative purposes only. Certain stock imagery © Getty Images.

Print information available on the last page.

ISBN: 978-1-9822-0756-4 (sc)
ISBN: 978-1-9822-0758-8 (hc)
ISBN: 978-1-9822-0757-1 (e)

Library of Congress Control Number: 2018907669

Balboa Press rev. date: 08/02/2018

CONTENTS

ACKNOWLEDGEMENTS

Thank you, Bear, for making it safe to let go of control. Thank you for telling me on our fourth date that I'm a writer, and thank you for reading every word I write. Your dedication to me is unmatched in my life thus far.

Thank you, Mama Llama, for believing I'm the best at everything. I love you so much.

Thank you to the amazing editor Katie Collins. Your guidance, your direction, your trust in me to say things the way I wanted to say them was unwavering.

Thank you, Ellen, for being my afternoon respite after long mornings of writing, and for inspiring me to be better.

Thank you, Mr. Mike Dooley, Nancy Levin, Reid Tracy, and Kelly Notaras. You truly are the driving forces behind finishing this book, whether you know it or not.

Thank you to my Peas. You know who you are.

Thank you Cerries, Keith, Heather, Shane, Mo, and Sarah for helping.

Thank you to Balboa Press and all of your support staff, especially Zara.

And most importantly, thank you, Abraham. You are my teacher. And even though you have to do what I say until you're a grown-up, I'm secretly learning to be a grown-up by being your mom. Thank you for choosing me.

Disclaimer

The events in this book are written from memory. Not all the events are in perfect sequence (though I tried my best), and occasionally I have compressed or combined the experiences to convey the substance of what occurred or what was said.

Although every experience in this book happened, it's important to note that I am not recommending you use *any* of them as a medical guide for infertility, pregnancy, or otherwise. The ideas and methods in this book are not suggestions or advice. There are very serious health risks involved in using any of the methods I used to get pregnant and to give birth, not to mention the very personal choices I made in my own treatment options. My incredible doctors researched and understood my specific biological makeup and prescribed a plan based on my specific needs and my requests. I am not a doctor, and I cannot know what is right for your body. My doctors are not your doctors. Therefore, my treatment and birthing plans are most certainly not right for you.

I have given the doctors and specialists nicknames in this book to protect their identity. I have also changed the names of many friends and relatives.

While I do hope you learn from this book, and I have gone to great lengths to ensure the information here about my diagnoses and treatments are up to date and factual, my descriptions are *informed at best* and should not be used as medical guidance in place of a doctor's advice.

INTRODUCTION

"All right! Time to make a baby!" I said to my husband.

"Yep! Baby making time!" he almost shouted.

I took off all of my clothes in front of the hotel room third-story window, drapes wide open.

"Babe! The window!" My husband pointed, eyes wide.

"It's okay. They're European. They probably do this all the time." I waved at some passersby. They smiled and waved back as if I was wearing clothes.

We were in Brugge, Belgium, a beautiful little city specializing in chocolate and lace. My husband, Phillip, and I were with his entire family on this once-in-a-lifetime trip to Europe, and we'd decided we were going to split off from the other twelve family members for a night or two. We considered it a one-year anniversary gift to ourselves, even though we'd been married a full fifteen months at that point. (Fifteen months is *way* longer than a year.) We ate soft pretzels and giant, smooshy waffles and drank beer that was chewier than the waffles; and, of course, we tried all different kinds of fudge.

And then, on a walk down a cobbled street back to our hotel in the middle of the afternoon, Phillip told me we should try to make a baby. Now, we'd discussed how fun it would be if we got pregnant during our trip to Europe, and I'd stopped taking birth control already, but babies were a fairly new topic of conversation for us. Though there was something very exciting about my own husband suggesting we go back to the hotel room and have sex for the sole purpose of attempting to make another human being. A little day drunk, a little love drunk, I agreed. "Yeah. Let's go make a baby."

He took off all of his clothes while I was waving to the strangers. The room was small, full of dark wood and bright white walls, and one entire wall was windows, so everything looked crisp. The sheets were very soft on our queen-sized bed—all white with a beautiful lace edge. We didn't waste too much time kissing or caressing. We jumped straight to the good part. No foreplay. No meaningful conversations. And while the sex was all fine and normal, there was this weird undertone that this was we-might-be-making-a-baby sex. I kept opening my eyes to look around the room so I would remember it. I wanted to be able to remember where we made our first baby.

"Do I have to do it at an angle?" he asked me, breathing heavily but with very little passion.

"No. Just do it, and then I think I hold my legs in the air afterwards and that's it," I answered mechanically.

"Okay. Makin' a baby," he reminded me.

"Yes." I remembered. "Here we go. Makin' a baby."

And here is where I tell you that, at twenty-seven years old, I didn't know how to make a baby.

I was married to my college sweetheart. I had a master's degree in school psychology. I could seamlessly navigate my way through the hills of Los Angeles where we'd moved four years earlier (and if you ask me, the hills of LA are way harder than marriage and a master's degree put together). I even knew how to oven roast a Thanksgiving turkey! (After I brined it!) But I didn't know how to make a baby.

Oh, I knew about which parts went where and which things swam toward which other things, and that when all the things combined … boom! Baby. But I thought that, when you did all those things on any given Tuesday in the middle of the afternoon in Brugge, two little purple lines would pop up in the indicator window of a pregnancy test a few weeks later, and then you'd cry and take pictures.

I had absolutely no idea there was more involved than "things combining."

My life up until that point had honestly been about as seamless as mastering my LA navigation skills. I had decided which college I was going to go to, I had applied and been accepted. I had decided I wanted to graduate college in three years. I'd done it. I'd decided I was ready to move across the country from my home state of Florida to live in a big city on the West Coast, and one day I'd packed my Ford Explorer and driven there. Boom. I lived in LA. I had decided who I was going to marry, he'd asked me, I'd said yes, and I had a husband.

Aside from a few very minor glitches in the matrix, my life had gone according to plan. And that's just the way I liked it. So, a few weeks after that afternoon in Brugge, when I took a pregnancy test and it was negative … I was very confused.

I had wanted a thing. I had done what it took to get the thing. And … I hadn't gotten the thing.

This was not fitting into my life equation.

My life equation had begun to take shape twenty years earlier. My beloved father passed away suddenly on a rainy weeknight. He was playing handball, as he often did after work, and we're told he collapsed on the handball court and died of a massive heart attack. When the phone rang, my mom and I were at home waiting for him as we did every night.

My dad knew everyone in the city of Akron, Ohio, where I was born, including the doctor who met my mother and me in a small, white waiting room of the hospital to tell us that my daddy was gone. He used those words: "He's gone."

When he said it, my mother's head flung back and hit the wall behind her chair as she emitted a blood-curdling scream. This was the worst, most unimaginable day of her entire life. My father had been her entire world. My mother and father were passionately in love up to the moment he died. They had been each other's worlds. Not to mention that I had no idea who would be my dad now.

The rest of that night was a blur. I don't know if my mother slept upstairs in the bed they had shared or who drove me home from the hospital. I only knew that I didn't like this feeling of being out of control, and there began my life equation: I would set my sights on things I could control, and then I would achieve them. I would stay safely in the circle of "it's easily attainable" and never again feel the fear or pain of being out of control. I avoided anything risky, anything that required a leap of faith. If it didn't fit my life's equation with 90 percent certainty, it didn't happen.

But at twenty-seven, I had no control over those two little lines on the pregnancy test. It was the first time in my life I had wanted something and I was not able take logical, life-equation steps to get it. And it was the most scared I'd been since the night I learned my mom and I were the only ones left. My mom had guided me through life, hiding the pain from me until I went to college. She never wanted me to feel that life-altering ache in my heart, and so, like any good mother would, she protected me from struggle and pain. And she protected me fiercely—so fiercely that I thought I'd created an infallible plan to live a peaceful, predictable life.

When I started writing this book, I tried to keep it light hearted and dance around the pain I felt every day as I waded through the experiences in the pages that follow. I wanted to protect you the same way my mother protected me from pain for as long as she possibly could. I wanted you to live my life equation: you get a book, you read the book, you feel better because it was the book you wanted it to be. In hindsight, I realize that my mom's best efforts to shield me from pain became my ultimate handicap as an adult (and also my greatest lesson). When life got challenging, when something looked like it might be a struggle, I turned and walked the other way. I moved to the area of the room where I could quickly and easily gain control and put things back together—neatly and in an order than made sense to me. I don't want to do that to you.

From my heart, I want you to know my struggle. I want you to recognize your own struggle, know that you are not alone, and know that there is an end to it. Pain and struggle are *required experiences* on Earth because, without them, put simply, we never find out what's on the other side of them. And, if you make it to the other side even just once, you realize that, like getting a tattoo, you immediately want to do it again. The journey hurts, but the other side is so, so sweet.

That all being said, this is a really freaking funny book.

I titled it *Finding Inner Peas* because laughter is my cure-all, even if it cures me for only a few seconds. While I found a new inner peace and acceptance during my infertility journey, I also took advantage of every excuse to laugh. I want you to laugh too. If we're going to find our own sense of "inner peas," sometimes it just has to start with laughter.

So, as you read along, laugh as if no one is watching! (Do not confuse this with "dance like no one is watching." That's an adorable metaphor for life, but unless you're completely alone, someone *is* watching you, and he's got a video camera in his phone. And you never *ever* want that boss or professor or grandparent to see that video of you dancing. For your own sake, dance as if people are definitely watching.)

PART 1

CHAPTER 1

Becoming an Adult

Moving to LA when you're twenty-three is kind of a big deal. When coworkers and friends in Iowa learned I was moving there, their eyes widened, and they breathed, "Where!"

I'd lean back casually. "Oh, to LA. You know. Whatevs." Then I'd dart my eyes to theirs so I wouldn't miss the jealous twinkle. This was incredibly satisfying for my ego. And that about sums up my twenties.

I'd moved to Iowa from Florida after college for a job, and my first address in Los Angeles was in North Hollywood, which automatically made friends and family assume I lived in Hollywood and not a semi-disgusting suburb of the valley that smelled like unkempt farm and transmission fluid. Truth is, I lived across the street from a KFC and a Goodyear tire store—a street with a couch in the alley on which random people were always sleeping and/or vomiting. The adult video store on the corner with the giant yellow "We have Paris Hilton" sign really classed it up though.

I had moved there to be with Phillip.

We met when I was nineteen, a sophomore at Rollins College in our home state of Florida. My boyfriend, Marcus, had just dumped me.

I was going to marry Marcus. And he dumped me.

That seemed like a terrible way to start our life together.

So, I did what any nineteen-year-old woman does. I cried and ate a lot ice cream. And when a cute, popular boy told me that his cute, popular roommate liked me and wanted to take me out to eat more ice cream, I eagerly obliged. Two cute, popular boys *and* ice cream? Okey dokey.

Tom was funny, with dreamy blue eyes, and was *waaaaay* cooler than I. I felt as though I had to impress him with my eyeliner and bad language. Tom asked me back to his place for some Jacuzzi tub fun. "Probably," I replied coolly, because I was awesome and not desperate.

So I bubbled in the hot tub along with cute popular boy, Tom, and another girl, drinking flavored alcoholic drinks out of bottles. Tom kept playing footsy with me. I giggled. It was obvious he was into me. This would go down in history as our "first date." Tom and I would become Mr. and Mrs. Tom. It was a really good night.

Until Tom got out of the hot tub and I was still playing footsy with—someone.

That was the first big surprise of our relationship. Because, as it turns out, I was playing footsy with cute popular boy, whose name you now know is Phillip.

• • • • • • • • • • • • • • • • • • •

After Phillip and I married in 2007, we felt as though it was time to turn the corner and start a phase of life that was more grown up, more goal oriented. (This was a stupid idea in hindsight, but whatever.) We were, after all, entering our late twenties, which meant our thirties were right around the corner, and no dignified thirty-year-old worked in a restaurant or as a teacher's assistant.

So we both got real jobs.

Phillip started working as a production assistant, and I got a job at a wealthy, hoity-toity private elementary school as a teacher. Meanwhile, I also went back to school and pursued a graduate degree in school psychology. You know why? Because it seemed like something I could do. I didn't actually want to be a school psychologist. But it was very impressive when my mom told people I was in grad school. I liked doing something I already knew I could do *and* it impressed people.

We packed lunches and adopted a dog, Charlie, who was a boxer from the rescue foundation up the street. Charlie immediately decided he trusted us and no one else, and he attempted to bite the hands and feet off anyone who came too close without permission (which we loved). We did our laundry at regular intervals and grocery shopped on Sunday mornings. We made our bed and designated an area within our apartment—not on the couch—for eating meals. Are you getting a sense of how grown up we were?

After a year of this, my husband called me at my fancy job and offered me the deal of a lifetime. He explained that his family had offered to move us to his hometown in Jacksonville, Florida, and help us get jobs, buy a house, and start a family. Our neighborhood would have sidewalks that weren't tagged with gang signs or phrases starting with the "F word."

This sounded way more grown up.

On our last night in LA, a friend invited us to a coffee house in the valley for a "final good-bye." When Phillip and I walked in, we saw twenty or thirty people we knew sitting at tables facing a stage meant for the local talent. I laughed as I greeted everyone, confused but happy to see them.

A crazy song came on, and my husband and I watched the words, "Phillip and Erin. This. Is. Your. ROAST." fly across a projector screen. Out of *nowhere,* one friend flung me over his shoulder and hoisted me onto the stage. Another taped cardboard flames to the back of my chair, and the coffeehouse roared with excitement to see the two of us completely flabbergasted and laughing our heads off, about to get our butts handed to us by the people we loved the most.

When the roasting was over, we went dancing in a bar so small, so hole-in-the-wall, it didn't even have a front door. It was the perfect ending to a perfect time in life. And it suddenly seemed viscerally wrong to drive away from it all.

In our empty kitchen, we both stared in opposing directions, mutual feelings of sadness floating around our bodies, until we eventually wandered off to our bedroom, which was now just a room because the bed was on the moving truck.

Our movers gave us a ten-day window to get to Florida (remember that the next time you're angry when the cable guy gives you a four-hour window), so we decided to take our sweet time as we drove from one end of the country to the other. We filled the hours by listening to comedy CDs—old Mitch Hedberg and Dane Cook—books on tape, and music. There wasn't as much talking as one would expect, and when we did talk we kept it light because, if we didn't, the weight of what was actually happening might encourage us turn the car around. During this drive to

Florida in Phillip's sporty little Audi A3, we were in limbo. Home wasn't behind us, and home wasn't in front of us.

Our first stop was Grand Junction, Colorado. It was January, but there wasn't any snow on the ground, which was fine by me. A rearview mirror "Jesus is my Homeboy" car freshener danced as we took the sharp turns through the mountains to get to the hotel I'd booked online. I chose hotels that allowed pets so Charlie would feel comfortable. I even knew where the closest animal hospital and veterinary clinic were in each city in case he got sick. I had each stop mapped with weather information and local food options, all highlighted and dog eared.

I know. It's a gift.

But the trip was cut short during our visit with one of my closest friends, Amy, in Iowa. The movers called to tell us they'd already arrived in Florida. They were five days ahead of schedule. "How does that even happen?" I shouted from the shower when Phillip told me.

We had to get home as soon as we could. And truth be told, we were five days into a ten-day trip, and we were already fairly sick of each other: "I'm pretty sure you missed the turn." I zoomed in on the map on my phone.

"No, I can go this way."

"Really? Because I'm physically *looking* at a map that says you cannot go this way."

"I can loop around."

"This map says you cannot do that."

"Well, that map doesn't know *everything*, Erin!"

"About mapping stuff it does!"

We stayed our last and sixth night in Nashville, and we hated each other that night. Our conversations were full of phrases starting with, "Well ..." split into three syllables that went up an octave at the end, and, "Maybe you should just ..." It was best to keep our mouths shut, which we finally decided to do around ten o'clock when all the divorce lawyers were probably sleeping. By morning, we would only have seven hours left to drive.

We pulled into Jacksonville around five in the evening and drove straight to my sister-in-law's house so we could sleep in a bed and start unpacking fresh the next day.

My sister-in-law Sharon was newly pregnant. A woman with properly coifed hair, enormous brown eyes with lashes curling up under her eyebrows, and the sweetest little southern button nose you've ever seen, Sharon is very practical. She doesn't use a whole lot of emotion, but she will open up her life and home to you at the drop of a hat if you need it.

I knew Sharon only as a family vacation acquaintance. She always called me on my birthdays, but we hadn't yet forged a true friendship.

The night we arrived, it was business as usual. Sharon fed her husband and kids dinner and walked around spraying air freshener to try to extinguish the dinner smell, which was, of course, bothering her pregnant sensibilities. Phillip and I slid right in to the goings-on in her house without feeling like a bother, and that was about the greatest thing I could ask for. I hated feeling like a bother.

She gave us the entire upstairs loft so we could spread out and feel secluded. The trip didn't yet feel over. I wasn't "home," so I didn't allow myself to have the your-entire-life-officially-changes-when-you-unpack-that-first-box feeling.

· ·

Moving into our house, which my in-laws had helped us buy, felt as grown up as I expected. It was a three-bedroom, two-and-a-half-bathroom craftsman-style home with a porch and a huge modern kitchen. We had found it months before on a visit home and bought it via email and phone calls. It had stairs and a second floor! This house was massive in comparison to our LA apartments, and our mortgage was the same as our rent!

When the movers were finished, we had a small kitchen table, an old, smooshy couch, a king-sized mattress, a few dressers, and a coffee table. It became very clear to me that we'd been living in a thousand-square-foot apartment for many years. Phil stood, forcibly happy, and took a deep audible breath with a big "Haaaa" at the end to convince me and himself that everything was all right.

For the first few weeks, our bedroom was empty, save for the mattress and the TV, which was propped up on a moving box. Phil usually fell asleep around ten. I, on the other hand, morphed into some sort of barn owl after we moved. I stayed up until all hours of the night, unable to go to sleep. Really there was nothing to wake up for.

At eleven thirty every night, *Will and Grace* came on. The show was so funny, and it became my solace. If I allowed myself to feel sad about being in a new place, it was because I knew that Jack would make me laugh soon. If I wanted to feel joy, I could just chuckle at the way Karen made Grace look stupid. *At least I have Will and Grace. At least I have this.*

To make matters worse, I didn't realize that the house was situated less than a mile from a railroad and that trains rolled through town about every hour at night. I lay in the dark listening to that train go by. If you've ever missed someone or someplace, then you know that the sound of a train whistle blowing through a darkened city is one of the most somber sounds the world can produce. It feeds sadness like a big old plate of fried chicken. It was a reminder that we had bought this house. We owned it.

I'd had a purpose in Los Angeles. Here, I just owned a house.

CHAPTER 2

Finding My Purpose

I now lived in the same city with a mother-in-law, a father-in-law, two sisters-in-law, their husbands, and four nieces and nephews. They'd lived there nearly all their lives by the time we joined them. I assumed I would immediately fit into my new extended in-law family. I figured, *If we're family, then family dinners and birthdays and holidays will feel like family. Like home.*

My in-laws were very welcoming, very kind, but the truth was, we simply didn't know each other. We'd never lived near each other, so holidays had been our only time together for the past seven years. My expectations were set to family mode, and my in-laws were busy accepting a virtual stranger at their dinner table.

To be fair, I was difficult.

I had weird eating habits they tried to accommodate. (First I was a vegan. After that, all I ate was meat.) I didn't drink sweet tea or soda. I wasn't a fan of college sports or politics.

My sisters-in-law offered me wine when I walked through the door at Phillip's parents' house because they knew I liked it. Then they'd get to work because they knew where everything was in the kitchen and exactly how to cook what their mom was working on. I felt uncomfortable not offering to help, but I didn't even know what to offer. When I did try to slide into the mix—chop carrots or dice a cucumber—I second guessed everything I did. I didn't know how they liked the salad to look. I didn't know if someone didn't want onions. So, usually, someone politely told me to set out the chips and salsa so I would have something to do. I would do that and sit back down again.

The half hour after dinner was worse. Everyone went right to work, sliding past each other and continuing the conversation as they set their plates in the kitchen, the leftovers on the kitchen table, and their glasses to the left of the sink. My sisters-in-law washed and dried and loaded the dishwasher in a practiced way while my mother-in-law enjoyed conversation with the men at the table. I was always on the verge of asking "How can I help?" while at the same time pushing myself to just do *something*. I was uber self-conscious. These weren't the creature comforts of home—or the family I'd grown over the years in LA, which would start a conga line through the kitchen to wash plates or simply get too drunk to do the dishes and leave them until morning.

"I know we're all going to get to know each other. I'm just worried it will never feel like family," I told Phillip on the way home one night. My eyes felt a little stingy, and I turned to look at the neat houses and the square yards rolling past us.

"Yeah. Family's tough, man. I have to get to know them all over again too," he replied. "I've been gone for ten years."

I decided I needed to find a job to give myself a sense of purpose.

All my contacts were in Los Angeles, so I was starting from scratch. I remember calling one school and starting my spiel with, "Hey, I'm Erin Salem, and my friend over at Empire High School recommended I call you! I'm new to—"

Before I even finished that first sentence, she interrupted, "I'm not hiring anyone. I'm not looking to hire anyone for a very long time."

I thought, *Oh really? Not for a very long time? You must be really good at your job and an incredible boss if you don't plan on needing any new staff members for a very long time. And when you do need new staff members because you are so rude to your current ones that they all quit, I will already have a job, so suck it!* But I just said, "Oh. Okay. Thank you."

Phillip was already working for his dad, so to try to find some normalcy in my routine, I did the laundry and watched a lot of the Food Network and made dinners. I searched desperately for my daily rhythm. Cooking became a survival mechanism, a complex activity I started at four o'clock in the afternoon just so I could focus on something I enjoyed that would take up time.

After about three months, when no one was interested in paying me to do anything with my fancy degree, I decided that cooking and managing the house and Phillip's life would be my new purpose. My life equation was not filling itself in, so I had to rush to fill it myself.

Phillip would come home to a hot meal and a clean house. Then I would get mad at him when he did the dishes or swept the floors because that was *my job*. It was all I had, so *don't do my job*.

Soon I decided I would take over the finances too. That lasted about a week, during which I confused our savings account with our checking account and couldn't figure out how to get my debit card to work. So I scaled back a bit and suggested I just take over the grocery budget. I determined a certain amount that we would spend each week on groceries and tried to enforce the new rule. This worked fine until Phillip bought groceries on the way home from work, prompting me to demand, "Well, how much did you spend? Did you save the receipt? Because it is my job is to take care of the grocery bills and make sure that we have the groceries that we need and that we don't go over budget!"

Then I made the rule that we would only use *cash* to buy groceries— the cash that I kept neatly in a little white envelope in the kitchen. Well, that didn't work because sometimes we bought groceries with a credit card and then tried taking the money out of the cash envelope to put it into the bank to pay the credit card to keep it balanced, but then we'd spend the cash on something frivolous because we had cash to spend.

Finally, I just gave up. I announced something like, "Well, I guess, you know, I will buy the groceries and then you can buy the groceries whenever you damn please, and we will spend however the fuck much we spend on groceries, and that is it."

That plan is still working.

• • • • • • • • • • • • • • • • • • •

It was about four months after we moved that I decided we needed to get a second rescue dog so Charlie wouldn't feel lonely in his new city (and so I would have something else to do). At eight months old, she was malnourished, and I could see every bone in her body. It took about two months to get her to a normal size and, by that point, we realized her brain was never going to get any bigger. Yes, she was a beautiful dog, but she was dumb as a bag of kibble. We named her Bella. Beautiful, stupid Bella.

After months of applying for jobs and trying to be the perfect housewife and raising two perfect dogs and eagerly waiting to see my in-laws at every family dinner, I noticed something: everyone around us had kids or was pregnant. They talked about their kids or their pregnancies. I tipped my wine glass and nodded knowingly ("Mmmhmm, oh yeah") during all of these conversations, but I didn't know what the hell anyone was talking about. Who cares if your kid switches from three naps to two? And why wouldn't you just give your kid the jarred baby food until she can eat ribs? Your child probably isn't sleeping because you're not *telling* him to sleep enough, that's how you do it. Does it really matter if your child is facing forward or backward in the car seat? He's in a *car seat*, isn't he? Get over it.

One night, I was sitting in my in-laws' kitchen while my mother-in-law was cooking something scrumptious. Sharon, who was a big six-months pregnant, told me I needed to hurry along and "catch up." "So when are y'all gonna get pregnant?" she asked. "This baby is going to need a playmate!" Sharon was pregnant with her third child, and Phillip's other sister, Margaret, was content with her two.

"I don't know," I said to her, feeling stupid for not having an answer. "We haven't really talked about it."

"Are you still on birth control?" she asked me.

"No."

"Well, good! Let's get crackin'!"

The truth was, we had been "crackin." After we decided to drunkenly *try* one afternoon in Brugge, and we didn't get pregnant, I'd been pretty upset about it. More upset than I should have been considering we'd had sex with the intention of trying to have a child *one time.* So we had continued "crackin" for the next few months. At this point it had been five months of "crackin'.

Five months. I hadn't realized we'd been without birth control for five months. It got me thinking. Sharon interrupted my introspection. "You start taking Robitussin yet?"

"No." I giggled. "Why?"

"It thins out your cervical mucus! Sometimes that helps women get pregnant more quickly." I stared at her. I could not believe she said cervical mucus *and* that I didn't know what that was. "You know—that mucus that comes out right before you ovulate?" she asked.

I did not know this mucus.

She could probably tell that I did not know this mucus because I must have looked as if she'd just described a body part that, for the first twenty-seven years of my life, I hadn't even known I had. "It's like stringy jelly. When you have that, you know you're ovulating!"

I was not positive what ovulating was.

She could tell that I was not positive what ovulating was because I agreed far too fervently.

"Ovulating is the time of the month the egg is ready to be fertilized and you can get pregnant. You can also tell if you're ovulating by how high up your uterus is. If you reach up and your cervix is pretty low, you're probably not ovulating. The higher it is, the closer you are to ovulating."

She could see the panic setting in on my face. There were times? Dates? I couldn't just get pregnant anytime I tried? I had to reach my hand up inside my vagina to measure how far up my uterus was while collecting jelly samples? "Or you can just get one of those pee-on-a-stick ovulation predictors from the drug store if you don't want to go reaching for your jelly," she said, temporarily interrupting my panic.

Huge sigh of relief there.

"Wow. Okay. What else do I need to know?" I asked, trying to sound interested but actually becoming desperate to find out what else I *didn't* know.

"Well, are you periods regular?" she asked me, crunching on chips and salsa.

"No, not really."

"That's okay. You could just be an irregular person, but you might want to let your ob-gyn know that. But I'd say that's it! You're ready!" She smiled. "Except don't have sex every day. That's not good for his sperm production."

Aaaaaaand ew.

I told you Sharon was practical.

But my brain was in high gear now. *I should get pregnant*, I thought. *I need to do it soon so my kid is the same age as hers.*

Aha! A purpose!

Trying to time the perfect meal, keep a spotless home, maintain a diligent grocery budget—none of these was really fulfilling. My life equation had been empty. But this! This filled a whole new equation! The *mom* equation: Want a baby, have the sex, become a mom!

That was a role that could be all mine. I was going to get pregnant. I had a plan. I was planning to get pregnant.

When Phillip finally overheard some of the conversation, he nosed in with a sort of curious and surprised look on his face. I got a little embarrassed that I was planning my pregnancy with his sister, but she jumped in and said, "Well, Phillip, you'd better get on it!" Her southern drawl helped make the situation feel lighter.

We were in the car about halfway home from dinner that night. Phil was driving, and I asked, "Well, do you want to just start trying?"

"Well, I guess *so!*" he said, as though it had mostly been decided for him.

"We should get one of those ovulation predictor tests."

"Yeah, I guess we should," he responded, having no idea what I was talking about but still being supportive.

At the next stoplight, I said, "So. I guess we are trying."

"Yeah. We are trying." Saying it out loud made us both smile. I could hear our thoughts shout *Yeehee, we are trying!* Somehow, saying it out loud made us both feel as if we were already pregnant.

CHAPTER 3

Not So Easy Peasy

On our way home that night, we stopped at a drug store so I could buy an ovulation predictor kit. I walked in through the automatic doors and immediately felt ridiculous. It was 9:30 on a Friday night, and I was shopping for an *ovulation predictor kit* while my husband waited in the car. Just a few short months ago, I would have been cooking my own meal on a grate at the cook-your-own-Asian-food restaurant in LA. My life there already seemed fuzzy in my memory.

I searched through all the different types in the family planning section and chose a generic brand because those stupid little pee sticks were expensive. I also grabbed a bottle of Robitussin in case that theory about the stringy jelly was true. As I approached the cashier, it seemed as though she already knew something about me—I was a little kid in a grown-up's body who was pretending she was about to try starting a family, but really she was just showing off for her friends because she needed attention. When the cashier turned to scan the test kit, I wanted to have a special moment with her. I wanted to squeal, "See what I am buying?"

And then she would say, "Yes! Wow! So you guys are trying?" Her face would be open and curious as she leaned toward me, thrilled to be my confidante.

And then I would say, "Yes! Maybe we'll even try this evening!" Then we would both giggle.

"Oh, that is so wonderful!" she would gush. "Well, congratulations to the two of you!" And I would float of out the drugstore after this magical moment feeling that it was all meant to be.

Of course, the way it actually went down was she said, "Fifteen ninety-nine," and then I gave her my credit card, and that was it.

When I got back into the car with the test kit in a little bag, the energy was like we'd just snuck out to buy condoms without our parents knowing. "What kind did you get?" Phillip asked.

"I don't know. The generic kind." I took it out of the bag and looked at the box while Phillip drove us the last few minutes home. I read the instructions without actually digesting any of the information. I stared at the box until we pulled into the garage and Phillip asked, "Are you going to pee on one?"

Once I *actually* read instructions, I realized that you have to pee on the stick in the morning. So that was when the peeing on the stick commenced.

I started each of the next thirty days by peeing on a stick at exactly the same time as the day before. When my hormones changed and my body was ready to produce an egg, the little tip of the stick would turn purple. I was incredibly dedicated to getting just the right amount of pee on each stick so as not to mess up the most important test I'd ever taken. Sometimes I peed into a little cup and then dipped the stick. Sometimes I peed directly onto the stick but not so forcefully that the pee splashed all over the stick or, worse, peed the stick right out of my fingers and into the toilet bowl. No, no. I was more respectful of a pee stick than all that. I was careful.

While the stick-peeing was taking place, I insisted that my husband and I have sex every other day just to be sure we didn't miss the ovulation day. (Life equation was want baby, *make* baby, become mom. I was already on to step two!) You would think this would be a party—a big sex party. You would think my husband would be chomping at the bit to get home every other day to try to make a baby. But, honestly, after about two weeks of sex every other day for the sole purpose of creating life, we were kind of sick of it. Bored, really. When sex is work, it's not that fun.

Neither is watching pee sticks.

Some days, the stick looked sort of purplish; some days it looked more like gray. One day, Phillip even walked in to congratulate me that the stick turned purple, but the truth was it just sat out on the bathroom counter too long, and the color wasn't accurate anymore. I peed and waited all thirty of those days until it became very clear to me that I was not achieving the results I'd hoped for. My pee sticks never made it to purple.

I was not, as it turned out, ovulating.

In June, a month after we decided to *actually try* instead of not not-trying, I felt that maybe my body wasn't working. Before we continued actually trying, I decided to call Sharon again and tell her that I'd been peeing on sticks and having sex every other day and things didn't feel right. Luckily, she took this all in with the scientific spirit I'd intended when I gave it to her. She bared no emotion and simply gave me the facts as she saw them, which was exactly what I needed. By the end of the brief chat, she and I agreed that I needed to see a gynecologist. Sharon recommended one.

Lady Doctor.

I followed the directions to Lady Doctor's office, and I walked into a huge, floor-to-ceiling glass lobby. The gal behind the reception desk took my picture with a polaroid, attached it to my file, and told me to wait. I guess they have so many patients that they have to take pictures to keep track of them all. That, or someone often tromps in to this gynecologist's office and poses as someone else to get an extra Pap smear.

Just as soon as I sat my bottom down in the chair, someone came out and called my name. Contrary to the implications of the photo taking, I was apparently their only visitor that day.

Lady Doctor came in the room shortly after I peed into a cup and allowed someone to weigh me while I wore a paper gown. Lady Doctor was short. She had cute blonde hair and crystal blue eyes. She didn't look at me as much as she looked at my paperwork. The little pleasantries weren't really that pleasant, but they weren't exactly unpleasant either, so I just continued making the small talk she seemed to enjoy.

"Isn't the weather gorgeous today?" she asked.

"It is," I responded. "My husband and I were thinking about taking a bike ride." *Unless bikes are bad for baby-making business, then we won't do it . . .*

"Oh, how nice. I see you live on the west side."

"Yes, we just bought a house there. We moved here from—"

"I just love the west side. If I could stand the commute I would live there." Keep in mind, our eyes really never met during this conversation until, "So, Erin, any questions for me?"

Hardly a segue, but I figured she's a doctor. Let me just lay it on her. "I've been trying to get pregnant for a few months and haven't been on birth control for a lot of months. I feel like something could be wrong here."

She continued looking at my paperwork, and I had to wonder if she was actually reading it or if she'd secretly snuck her Kindle into the stack so she didn't have to miss a moment of the Harlequin Romance novel she was into. Finally, when I finished talking, she offered me an easy smile. "It's nothing to worry about," she said, sort of as if I hadn't really said anything. "Lots of girls don't start a regular cycle after birth control pills for months and months."

I appreciated her comparing me to "lots of girls," but I still felt like something wasn't right. "Is there something I can take to help get regular periods and ovulate? I don't think I'm ovulating."

"No," she replied, writing notes on her little Lady Doctor pad. "Not really. But let's give it time. I'm sure everything will start back up."

You know, like a car.

"Well, can we investigate anyway?" I asked. She smiled placatingly at me, as though I was asking her to check *one more time* that there were no monsters under the bed.

"I don't think it's necessary," she said. She shut me down four or five more times and then, being that she herself was a visible six months pregnant, cheerfully waddled her big-ass round belly full of baby into the next room.

Bitch.

I thought about leaving an anonymous threatening note using letters cut from the five-year-old magazines in the exam room basket, but I decided it was probably time to start a phone call parade instead. I began calling Lady Doctor's office incessantly, reiterating every symptom I had in hopes that they would take me seriously, or, like in an episode of *House*, someone would suddenly and angrily stumble upon a diagnosis. (I've got it! Her uterus is upside down! Let's flip it!)

I found one nurse, Belinda, in the office who consistently called me back. I inundated that poor woman with messages for a week. I knew the automated voice system path straight to her inbox better than I knew my debit card code. My strategy was to be sickeningly nice. I was so nice I had to curse at kittens when I hung up just to even out the Universe. Belinda pretended to care about my concerns and finally decided to do something so that "Salem" didn't pop up on her caller ID anymore. She ordered blood work.

Fine. Blood work. It's a start.

I hung up the phone and called Sharon from my kitchen to tell her they were going to run blood tests.

"This is a good thing," she assured me, her voice briskly confident. "Finding out what is going on now is so much better than waiting."

"Uh huh," I said, totally unconvinced.

"It is. Once we've got an understanding of what's going on, we can deal with it. You know, I had trouble getting pregnant with my first two. I had an issue with my endocrine system, and all it took was a simple pill to fix it. The condition is called PCOS. So if you have that, it might be an easy fix!"

When I hung up the phone, the house was quiet except for Charlie and Bella's snores. Phillip was at work, so to distract myself from my obsessive worries, I buried my head in my computer researching PCOS. It stood for polycystic ovarian syndrome. What I read was confusing and conflicting, and even though I was taking notes, I wasn't entirely sure how to tell if I had PCOS or what it even meant.

I'd recently taken a small work-from-home administrative position, so after about an hour of "research," I closed out all my search browsers and opened my email. It was easy work and didn't interrupt my constant need to call Lady Doctor's office with the hopes that *someone somewhere* was going to figure this out for me.

Two days later, I arrived at the blood lab at 6:45 in the morning. The doors would open at seven, and I was first in line. My paperwork was neatly organized and within easy grabbing reach inside my bag, and I'd been fasting since eight o'clock the night before. I was ready.

I stepped into a large waiting room with about nine other people after signing in. Several moments later, I was called to window two, and a woman in scrubs sat across from me confirming my address and insurance information. As always, I tried to make small talk. And as per my experience with medical personnel up to that point, she wasn't really interested.

She clicked on her keyboard until all the fields on her screen were filled in, and then she told me to take a seat in the next hall over. I walked back, farther into the building, down a hallway until I saw a set of chairs. I sat down, nervously looking around to see if I was doing this right, when I saw a phlebotomist (this is a fun word, so say it out loud anytime you read it) in the first stall. I peered down the hallway to see seven or eight stalls all in a row, presumably each filled with a phlebotomist. I watched the one near me as she set up a bunch of vials on a small table next to a tall, cushy chair. One. Two. Three. Four …

What Belinda had failed to mention was that I would be having ten vials of blood taken in one morning. *Ten!* She also hadn't mentioned that I would have to take a glucose test. The long and short of this test is that a phlebotomist takes your blood and then hands you one of those short, fat plastic bottles of sugary drink with a foil cap, just like the ones they used to hand out at summer camp. It tasted as bad as it did when we were in camp, but none of us campers said anything back then because … *just keep giving us sugar!* Then, I had to wait in the hallway for an hour so the sugar could swim around my body and make me feel sick. I had no idea what this had to do with getting pregnant. Finally, another phlebotomist took one last eleventh vial of blood and sent me on my weary way. I felt nauseous, had the world's worst headache, and just wanted to sleep without ever waking up. At about three o'clock that afternoon, it became crystal clear that Belinda was punishing me with a glucose test.

It took two weeks for the test results to come in, and when they did, I took the first appointment I could get to see stupid, cute little pregnant Lady Doctor again. She told me my hair looked nice and that my levels were only one or two points off and that she really didn't see any major problems (in one breath). She recommended I see a reproductive endocrinologist and get a "professional opinion." (So, I'm not really sure what that made Lady Doctor over here, but whatever.)

When I had sex with my husband for the purpose of getting pregnant and I did not, in fact, get pregnant, I felt uncomfortable. But when Lady Doctor told me I needed to see a reproductive endocrinologist, I felt shame. My one job was to make eggs in my body and grow them into babies.

Biologically that was truly my one job. Could I not do that? Without medical intervention? It seemed like a huge jump from a regular doctor to a specialist. There was now a fracture between the person I always thought I was meant to be and the person it actually turned out that I was. And none of it fit my life equation.

I'm a woman who can't get pregnant without a doctor's help. I'm a woman who needs help being a woman.

The realization that I needed a reproductive endocrinologist left me depressed. *There is something wrong with me.*

It was after I learned our insurance didn't cover any part of infertility treatments that I began to feel panicked. *There is something wrong with Florida.*

Most insurance companies have a lot of rules, usually consisting of deeply researched ideas similar to, "I can't stop writing the ticket once I start because I already started writing it." I knew that women could spend upwards of $40,000 trying to get pregnant and, having been in charge of the grocery budget at one time, I knew we did not have an extra $40,000. And now that I had some investigatory blood work done, insurance companies everywhere raised their red flags and called each other to whisper, "Don't cover Erin for anything. She just wants to steal all of your money and give it to a reproductive endocrinologist for no good reason. She's that kind of girl."

At that time, health insurance required you to have what's called an "infertility rider." That was an additional insurance plan—like a side of French fries—to our regular health insurance that would help pay for some parts of this journey we were about to embark upon. The only reason we got the infertility rider at all was because, after seven or eight tries, I finally figured out how to answer every question the man/woman in a foreign country with a decidedly "American" accent asked me.

"Do you have a diagnosis?"

"No."

"Have you had testing done?"

"No."

"How long have you been trying to get pregnant?"

"A year."

"Do you ever smoke or drink?"

"No."

Most of my answers were straight-up lies, but after making enough of those calls, I said what I needed to say.

The weeks between learning I might need extra help getting pregnant and actually getting to see a doctor who might help me, I worked. I worked a lot. I couldn't spend any time being anxious or frustrated about the fact that my ovaries were on strike.

Phillip and I spent most of the time falling in love with new TV shows like *Dexter* and *Sons of Anarchy*. One day was pretty much a carbon copy of the next: wake up, Phillip goes to work, Erin works out to a DVD upstairs, Erin goes to work downstairs, Erin cooks dinner, Phillip comes home, Erin and Phillip and the dogs watch TV, and then bed. Oh, and sex happened a normal amount and no longer felt forced or stressed, although we both probably thought whenever we had sex: *What if all our worry is for nothing and we're actually about to conceive a baby right now?*

And when we finally learned our insurance would go into effect, I got an appointment with the reproductive endocrinologist five days later. I trotted in, all prepared with my calendars, my lists, my blood tests, and my research. I'd already sent along my blood work from Lady Doctor, but I had copies with me just in case.

We were sent to sit down in a beautiful little room called "Telluride." Every room in the infertility office was named after one of the doctor's favorite vacation spots. Photos of the doctor and his family vacationing in Telluride, Colorado, lined the walls. Beautiful, hard-copy books sat on the table. Phillip chose *Basics to a Woman's Uterus* and I chose *Good Calories, Bad Calories*. We sat reading and nervously awaiting the doctor when a jolly, middle-aged woman flounced in. "Erin?"

I looked around, wondering if someone else in the room might have my name because she seemed incredibly happy to see whoever Erin was.

"Erin? You're Erin, right?"

"Um, yes, ma'am?" I panicked. Had I met her during a drunken football game?

"Oh, great! Hi! I'm Pam!"

Pam was slightly overweight. She had brown-and-gray hair and a smile that made you wonder if she was always at a party. Her voice was a little scratchy but kind of sing-songy. Oh, and it turned out that Pam didn't know me after all. She was just really energetic and had discovered, when she read my chart, that we lived only two blocks from each other. We talked about that for fifteen minutes. Fifteen minutes! I did my best to follow her train of thought and stay interested in our geographical proximity while my brain screamed, *Hello, Pam! Can you tell me what's wrong with me? Why can't I make a baby or an egg? Can we talk about that?*

"So, anyway, you probably want to know what's going on," Pam said with a laugh. Phillip's eyes met mine, and I almost giggled at the absurdity.

"Yeah, Pam, that'd be great."

"Okay, well, let's just get to it. We went through your blood work numbers. You're prediabetic."

Yeah. Let's pause. Let's take that in. Let's just take. That. In. A woman who was just giving me times and dates for the next German-American Club get-together has now announced with her next breath that I'm prediabetic. First of all, I'm Lebanese, and second of all, I'm what?

"I'm what?"

I started crying. It wasn't a hysterical cry. It was the cry you cry when your dog starts pooping out string or stuffing and you start to panic, wondering if the dog is okay and which decorative pillow has been destroyed in the house. It was a deep breath, hold-on-for-what's-coming cry.

"Prediabetic. I know. Crazy right?"

"Yeah, Pam. That's pretty crazy," Phillip said.

"Well, it gets crazier. You have polycystic ovarian syndrome. Or you can call it PCOS."

Oh, boy. Sharon had told me about that syndrome once. I'd already Googled that syndrome! I started to breathe faster, relieved but panicked at the same time. Here was the answer to my question on a silver platter, and I kind of wanted to send it back and order the soup.

Pam didn't really explain what any of this meant. Well, that's not true. I paid no attention to Pam while she explained what *all* of this meant. I felt numb, as if I were traveling down a tunnel of people who were staring at me and reaching out to touch my hair even though *I just asked them not to.*

A few moments later, the doctor, a kind-eyed guy who could not have been much older than I, walked in and sat down. I recognized his brown mop of hair and dark eyes from the pictures of him in Telluride lining the room. He was from New York (which I'd learned from Pam during our geography lesson) and wore a gold chain around his neck. Not like a mafia gold chain. A modest one that said, "I'm from New York, but I'm not going to overdo it." I started calling him Dr. New York in my head.

"So, have we gotten this conversation started?" he asked.

"I'd say so," I said.

As Dr. New York spoke, my husband sat next to me, sort of silently taking it all in. I say "sort of" silently because he cleared his throat and shuffled in his chair a lot. I could tell he didn't know what to do. Sometimes he awkwardly touched my shoulder in an attempt to "comfort" me, but it felt more like a first date touch than a husband touch, and I wasn't very comforted.

We spent two hours in that room with Dr. New York and Pam learning about PCOS and the hormones related to sugar (glucose) in the blood that cause it. (Ironically, Pam let me keep *Good Calories, Bad Calories*, since it was all about sugar. My husband had to leave *Basics to a Woman's Uterus* behind.)

Here's a little bit of what I learned: polycystic ovarian syndrome can be hereditary but often isn't, and almost 10 percent of women have it during their reproductive age. Ovaries make a bunch of hormones, but the two lady hormones that grow eggs and then send them on down the pike to the uterus are estrogen and progesterone. Ovaries also make a little bit of testosterone so women can grow healthy bones and feel energized (testosterone also provides about two hundred other benefits). Women with PCOS don't make quite enough of those lady hormones, and they make a little too much testosterone. Too much testosterone causes weight gain, acne, facial hair, hair loss, depression, infertility, and a whole boatload of other issues. I wasn't overweight, had no facial hair, and had experienced no hair loss, but I had struggled with acne and depression at different points in my life.

And now, it seemed, I was also struggling with infertility.

You see, our ovaries grow these little fluid sacs each month call follicles. These little guys keep our eggs safe and warm until our lady hormones tell the follicles to open up and let the eggs slide from the ovary, down the fallopian tube, and into the uterus. When women don't have enough estrogen and progesterone, nobody calls the follicles to tell them to release the eggs (which is why I peed on a stick for so long and never got the purple you-made-an-egg signal). Since they never get the call, the fluid filled sacs just keep on growing and growing. On an ultrasound, they look like a string of peas lining the uterus. It's now that the doctor will call your ovaries polycystic—*poly* meaning "many" and *cystic* meaning "fluid-filled sacs."

So why, oh why does my body make too much testosterone and not enough lady hormones? This is where things got interesting and borderline weird.

When a woman eats sugar (glucose), the sugar knocks on the pancreas's door and asks if the insulin can come out to play. Insulin jumps in the car and drives around the bloodstream, collecting up all the sugar, and delivers it to the cells and helps them to deal with that sugar in the appropriate ways like sticking it in the pantry for later when we need to use it for energy. But women with PCOS have cells like a petulant teenager. When insulin shows up to deliver glucose to the cells, they're, like, "Nah. I can do this myself. I don't need you bringing glucose to me." So the insulin just leaves the glucose on the cells' doorsteps and drives off. The cells can't absorb all of the glucose alone before it drifts back off into the blood stream, though. The glucose is lost and confused, and so it takes an Uber back to what it knows: the pancreas.

"Knock-knock-knock. Can we get some more insulin?"

The pancreas is a super nice guy, and even though he *just gave you insulin*, he gives you some more. That insulin drives back to the cells with the sugar, and now the cells pretend they don't even know insulin anymore! So insulin goes back home, but not before it gives the cells the finger and says, "The next time you need me to deliver you sugar, you'll be sorry. I'm not coming out!" Insulin then starts spreading rumors about the cells on Facebook.

This is called insulin resistance. Since the cells won't take the insulin's help to process the sugar, there's extra sugar everywhere. Once that happens enough times, the pancreas gets way too tired to produce more insulin, and a person will become prediabetic and, later, diabetic.

How does this relate to lady hormones and testosterone?!

Well, when there's a bunch of insulin just floating around the lazy river of the bloodstream, and the sugar is along for the ride, the body experiences inflammation. Because there are now all these red flags about the insulin and glucose, the ovaries are like, "Well, obviously you don't need to worry about getting pregnant right now. You've got bigger fish to fry. I'll just slow up on the progesterone and estrogen until you get that mess under control."

Here's the kicker: insulin just *happens* to trigger ovaries to release more testosterone. Which normally would be totally fine if we aren't already dealing a mass influx of insulin!

In essence, we were told that strawberry jam and fruity drinks made me infertile, and I would have to cut it *all* out if I wanted to have a family. I would have to eat protein, fat, and starch-free vegetables. I would need to take a prescription to help continuously eliminate sugar from my body. I would have to stop exercising and start meditating.

Now, when someone tells you that you should give up sugar, you assume they mean Butterfingers and Cinnabons. But my doctor gave me a list of things I could eat that paled in comparison (at least in desirability) to the things I could not eat. "Fertility Diet" was the title on top of the Xeroxed paper I received. It included things like nuts, lettuce, and entire sides of beef. What I could *not* eat included cheese, bread, potatoes. rice, pasta, and *fruit*. I would need to stick to foods that my body couldn't possibly confuse with sugar and accidentally request an insulin response. Without sticking to this diet, my body would start the whole insulin response over again. And if that happened, it would take at least a month to calm everything down. Long term, if I didn't change the way I ate, Dr. New York gave me ten years at most before I developed full-blown diabetes, pregnancy notwithstanding.

I'm not going to lie. I considered giving up right then and there.

Dr. New York gave me some literature to read along with the food list and scheduled an appointment for an ultrasound. We left with our stack of papers and got into the elevator. Phillip and I stood silently beside each other, waiting to reach level one.

Finally. "I don't want to be sick," I whispered. "I don't want to have diabetes. I don't want to change my whole life."

"I know, babe," he said and wrapped his arms around me just as the elevator doors opened. He didn't let go. He let the doors close. I tucked my arms in to his chest and let him take complete control of the hug, wrapping me all up so I could close my eyes and breathe.

CHAPTER 4

Peanuts? Yes Peas

I allowed myself to feel sorry for only about an hour before I kicked back into action. Life equation now looked like this: Want baby, cut out all sugar before making baby, make baby, become a mom.

It was late afternoon, and we stopped at the pharmacy to get the prescription for the sugar-removing medication called Metformin. They were inexpensive, which somehow made me feel better because this meant they'd been around long enough to earn a generic brand. On the way home, Phillip flipped through radio stations and tapped the steering wheel until he asked, "Do you want to just pick up dinner? Let's give ourselves a break and get take out."

"Yes," I nodded. "Hell, yes. I'm not cooking right now. I don't even know what I can cook or how to cook it."

We walked into our house, both feeling a little out of our bodies, and the dogs greeted us without any reservation. *You guys don't even know I can't process sugar, do you?* I thought.

Phillip handed me a sushi menu from the menu drawer in the kitchen, his brow wrinkled. "I don't know. It seems like you can order stuff off of this menu, but I keep looking at the fertility diet list of foods and …"

I took the menu and scanned it, cross-referencing the list on the counter. Rice? No. Raw fish? Yes. Salad? Maybe, unless there was sugar in the ginger dressing. Tempura-fried anything? Nope. Seaweed salad? Yes. But who wants seaweed salad?

By the time Phillip got home with the take-out order, my dinner looked like a hundred little bites of random fish and pieces of very specific vegetables in a box. I sat with Phillip at the coffee table in the living room eating one bite of fish and one bite of seaweed salad and one bite of steamed broccoli, watching Phillip eat his spicy tuna handroll. I felt as though something had been taken away from me. *No way*, I thought. *I can't do this.*

But if I wanted a child—and I did, desperately—I had to. So I took my fertility diet list with me everywhere and constantly checked it to see what I could and couldn't eat. I could eat nearly nothing in restaurants, so going out with friends sucked because I had to grill the server about how the meat was cooked, whether or not there was sugar in the marinade, if there was breading, if a vegetable was fried, or if there might be some sort of dried fruit hiding in the salad.

At one point during the crazy restrictive diet period, we took a weekend trip out to Vegas. I asked the server if the corned beef hash came with potatoes (because potatoes are a starch and I couldn't eat starches). She nodded. I then asked if the potatoes were mixed in, or if they were big chunks like home fries that I could easily pick out. She told me they were big chunks, so I went ahead and ordered a large portion, excited to be able to eat something delicious that followed all the rules of the diet. You guessed it—there were small bits of potato mixed in to the whole dish.

I stared at it, so freaking frustrated, for several minutes before I carefully, angrily picked out all the little potatoes and piled them next to the little fruit cup that came with the corned beef hash, and by the time I had a plate of food I could eat without threatening my ability to *make another person*, everyone else at the table was finished with breakfast and I had to pack mine up to go. Nothing about eating was fun anymore.

Meanwhile, the Metformin made me feel sick and uncomfortable every morning. I woke up completely aggravated with the lack of food options all day in between running to the bathroom in order to experience *more* diarrhea. Oh, the diarrhea. That was a fun little addition to the misery of adapting to the medication. Let me tell you how pleasant I was to be around.

Every day, I got up, drank my coffee with no sugar and no cream, ate my hard-boiled egg and bacon, and went to work in our home office until shortly after lunch (which was mostly salads with chicken). I was supposed to be meditating, but do you know how boring that is?

So instead of meditating, I researched. Over the course of one month, I earned my PhD in Google Doctor School specializing in PCOS and prediabetes. I researched until it was time to begin cooking dinner (meat and more lettuce) and then often spent an hour (or three) after dinner researching more. "Aha! This woman cured her PCOS with cinnamon! I need to eat more cinnamon!"

In that time, I also saw that my work-from-home job would be imperative to paying what I knew would be expensive, open-ended fertility treatment bills. Without it, we would have to start selling off my husband's sneaker collection. And while I'm pretty sure we could have earned enough to pay for the entire experience with those shoes, my husband might also lose his will to go on living without them, so it just wasn't an option. I would *not* be a single mom.

A few days after the initial diagnosis, I had my follow-up appointment with Dr. New York. This time we were escorted to a room called ... some South American city with a name I couldn't pronounce. But the colors in the room were beautiful, and the pictures of Dr. New York and his family living it up were hilarious. In one of them, he held up maracas while his wife pretended to blow into some kind of bright-red wooden horn. In another, he held up colored beads, and his wife's head was flung back in hysterical laughter. The pictures felt contrary to the situation.

It was here I would be discussing my options for fertility treatments with the doctors and eating dry roasted peanuts (because they were my only approved snack). I came prepared with the peanuts. I also came prepared with a lot of questions. How did I get this syndrome? How long had I had it? I knew my sister-in-law had children, but would I be able to? Were there varying degrees of PCOS that caused some women to give up hope? How long would I have to eat peanuts for every snack? And was there even a remote possibility that I was doing more harm than good to my body by eating all this meat and fat?

Dr. New York entered with Pam, and they both shook Phillip's hand. Pam immediately complimented my shoes and my necklace and laughed about the time she lost a necklace while swimming in a lake. She'd looked for it with goggles which, of course, wouldn't work because lakes are murky. Dr. New York smiled while she rambled and eventually made eye contact with me, asking, "Can I get you some peanuts?"

I held up my peanut jar. "I brought some!" I smiled.

Dr. New York began answering my questions and, as it turned out, he knew more than Google, which was reassuring. He told me PCOS is not really a diagnosis but a set of symptoms, some of which I had and some I didn't. Some women with PCOS don't even have any symptoms.

He told me this was probably hereditary, I would definitely be able to have children with help, and some of the lifestyle changes I was applying might have to be lifelong. The diet would definitely not affect me negatively because I would eventually be able to add back some of the other food groups. For now, we were being strict solely to help get me pregnant. He said the degree to which a woman experiences the symptoms of PCOS depended a lot on lifestyle and diet.

He talked slowly but not so slowly that he made me feel as if *I* was slow. I could tell as he spoke that he knew there would never be enough answers for me even if he brought in a white board and some of the chicks from *The Price is Right* to diagram everything out for me and dramatically point at it all. The truth was, I wasn't really seeking the medical whys, even though from the outside that was what it seemed. I was seeking the hows. How were we going to overcome this?

I'd never met a "what" I couldn't "how." Between our cross-country move, my lack of meaningful work, and now infertility, I felt worthless. Over and over again, I'd been faced with "whats" I couldn't "how," and now I was going to have to start relying on *other* people to help me "how." And other people are often a letdown. They sometimes don't show up, and sometimes they die really suddenly.

Dr. New York didn't psychically answer the lunch dates part. He worked with Pam and another nurse, Winnie, to complete an internal ultrasound to confirm my PCOS. When the picture of my uterus came up on the screen and my ovaries soon took center stage, I could see them: they really did look like strings of pearls. Cysts in my ovaries made them look like oysters with pearls.

He then suggested I have a hysterosalpingogram (HSG) test. Basically, this is when another person looks inside your body to see if the tubes that lead from your ovaries to your uterus are open. There's no sense spending a bunch of money to get the eggs crackin' if the plumbing's all blocked up. (I think that's a line from one of Will Smith's early albums.) They fill up your uterus with squid ink or whatever and watch a TV screen to see if the ink will flow freely all the way through the tubes. Dr. New York made sure to tell me that this was not a mandatory test, but he strongly suggested it. So, I made the next appointment at an outpatient surgery center. *HSG, here I come.*

CHAPTER 5

The Kind of Mom I Can Be

I was hyper focused on getting pregnant now. Thus, between the biological clock and my need to overcome this obstacle, my conscious brain turned off, and I became a pregnancy superhero, complete with the cape, willing myself to get pregnant in a single bound (but with adorable hair).

Because I was so focused, I didn't give much thought to the result of getting pregnant: you know, a kid? I rarely floated off into daydreams about what motherhood would be like. For whatever reason, my daydreams included only my child being an infant for a couple of days. Then, suddenly, he or she was going to be old enough to watch TV and movies with me and go for walks and just generally hang out. I pictured getting up, having coffee (with cream and sugar), and walking to the front office where my kid would simply entertain himself while I worked. That would be life.

And, if you have a kid, you're laughing.

So most of my fantasies were about *being pregnant* rather than having an actual child. I perfected the vision of me walking into my ten-year high school reunion—balloons and confetti in the old gym—being round and pregnant in an adorable red maternity dress. I was nervous about attending my ten-year reunion because, well, I used to live in LA. Now I lived back in Florida. I used to be in graduate school and work for movie companies and do amazing things like camping and going to concerts in my spare time. Now I was lucky if the movie I wanted to see came to the city I lived in. I didn't have anything to show for the life I was currently living, so if

I showed up as just me, no one would be impressed. But if I showed up pregnant … well, that … *that* would be something.

Then there was the belly-touching fantasy—like my belly was a novelty item that I could buy at Brookstone's and show off and let people oogle. "Ooo! She has one!" I envisioned walking through the grocery store and stopping at every third or fourth cereal box to let someone else feel the baby kick. I imagined complaining about how uncomfortable I was and thanking every Tom, Dick, and Harry who let me go first in the buffet line because they totally understood I was eating for two.

And, of course, the labor fantasies—breathing, heaving, holding onto banisters. Rocking on all fours or shoving someone out of my way as I walked through a heavy contraction. And then, pushing and shouting and struggling to bring life through me and out into the world. Everyone would congratulate me and shower me with loving words. The room itself would swell with pride. Because, in *my* labor fantasy, pain wasn't involved.

I never considered what kind of *parent* I would actually be. My parents were relaxed parents, partly because my dad was so experienced. He had six kids before me with his first wife, and I was, to put it nicely, an afterthought. Mom and dad never intended to have kids, and my mom completely trusted him, so she didn't need to panic the way a new mom often does. They treated me like a regular old member of the family starting the day I was born. They took me out to dinners from the time I was six months old. Not IHOP dinners. Fancy dinners. White tablecloth dinners. There were no chicken nuggets or mac 'n cheese on those menus. My parents ordered me angel hair pasta slathered in olive oil and fresh herbs (which I twirled using a fork and spoon) and perfectly roasted lamb shanks. I was just a small adult who went along with them everywhere.

But beyond being very chill, my parents were magical when I was little. Around my fifth year of life, my dad came home from work early on a rainy day. He flung the front door open and, instead of his usual waltz straight into my mother's arms, he frantically scooped me up. "Rainbow!" he screamed. My mother hurriedly got my shoes and coat while my dad continued ranting and raving, telling me to hurry up or we'd miss it. I was excited, though I didn't quite know what a real rainbow was yet. He tossed me into the front seat of his big old brown truck because, in 1985, car seats weren't a big deal. He drove like a bat out of hell, pointing and yelling, "Do you see it? Do you see the rainbow?" I looked and I looked, smiling, laughing, searching. Finally, I saw it. *Ooooh*, I thought. *It's the colors in the sky.* I was thrilled when I could finally join my dad in his excitement, really join him because I saw it.

We continued driving down a long dirt road, staring at the rainbow. I still, to this day, don't know where that road was. I remember it like one of those roads on *Dateline* they film to show how "isolated" it was where they found the body. Cornfields or something similar lined both sides, and trees lined the horizon, but all in a blur as the truck lumbered along. Finally, my dad yelled, "Ooooh, *no!* It's fading! We have to find the end!" I didn't know what the end was. And I'm not even sure if he ever told me. He just started driving faster. He was smiling with his whole face, and I started chanting, "Faster! Faster, Daddy! Don't miss it!" Eventually he pulled the car to the side of the road and frowned. "Aww. It looks like it's gone. It's gone. Wanna get ice cream?"

That was how they raised me. They wanted to see the world through my eyes. They wanted to experience it all with me for the first time and show me just how beautiful all these things in life were. "Just look at this rainbow that has been created for us to see!" I can hear them saying.

My parents made parenting look easy. That was the kind of parent I wanted to be now.

I didn't go visit my dad's grave until I was about twenty-five, and I've actually never been since. It started out because I was scared, and now it's because I live hundreds of miles from his final resting place. When I was little, I would just send letters with my mom for her to leave at his grave. One day, probably unconsciously, I drew a rainbow and gave it to her to "give" to him after he died. It wasn't my favorite, and I chided myself for sending something that wasn't my best work to my dead father.

Some years later, I was acting in a college show called *Blithe Spirit* about dead people coming back and communicating with the living. As research, my castmates and I visited a medium. She agreed to explain to us how she did her work but prefaced the visit with a stern "I'm not doing any readings." We sat in her elaborately decorated house with vaulted ceilings and lots of dark wood. She sat on the white-carpeted floor of her living room with the cast of the small show, despite the white leather couches, and answered our questions about how she came to do what she does. Her long black hair clung to her cream cardigan as she told us the story of her first experience communicating with the dead when she was young. In her ethereal voice, she described her dead brother standing in the kitchen. She described talking to him, and later talking to her grandfather. She didn't do any convincing. She didn't *need* to convince us. We just believed her. I waited and watched, knowing that Dad was going to annoy her until she said something. He wouldn't pass up this opportunity. Finally, her eyes turned to me.

"I talk to my dad all the time," I said without her asking me any questions. The room fell quiet as she continued to stare at me, just stare. I waited until I got too uncomfortable to let the silence linger. "He's here, isn't he?" I asked.

She smiled and nodded. "He says, 'Thanks for the rainbow.'"

●●●●●●●●●●●●●●●●●●●●

A few days after Dr. New York suggested it, Phillip drove me to the HSG test. I was told it should be a quick procedure at an outpatient surgery center. Our insurance company agreed to pay for part of this eight-hundred-dollar day, and we were ever so grateful to them for finding it in their hearts to do *their jobs*.

I asked a few times if the test hurt, and everyone assured me it wasn't so bad. "Just a little cramping sometimes." So while I sat in an individual waiting room, wearing an open-back gown, I texted my husband out in the lobby and read trashy websites about addicted celebrities and their pets. Feeling no pressure. The curtain separating my room from the next room was camouflaged and was decorated with a picture of a deer. Stay classy, Florida.

A sweet little prepubescent nurse called me into the "surgery" room, which happened to be the brightest room in the world. I lay down on the metal table, and the real nurse came in to do the procedure.

"Hey girl!" she said. "She" was Winnie. I liked her. She worked in Dr. New York's office, was very funny, and made uncomfortable processes bearable and almost fun. She was the one who had given me my first internal ultrasound to confirm I had PCOS and, when she did, she announced I had the cutest little uterus in town, a beautiful string of "peas" (cysts), and then remarked that my cervix looked like a smiley face.

She even offered to let my husband see my smiling cervix. He looked at me like a child who stares at his mom after his best friend asks him if he can sleep over: "Can I, Mom? Can I?"

Winnie chatted and giggled with me as she set up her tools for the HSG. "... and they forgot the cheese! After all that, they forgot the cheese!" The other nurses were laughing at Winnie's story too. I stared at the television screens to my right, where my uterus would soon star in its own show. I waited to see the ink injected and the tubes wide open. Winnie apologized that the speculum was so cold. (For the men here at the party, these are long, skinny tongs they use to open a woman's vagina during medical exams, so congratulations on having a penis.) She began the procedure, and all the other nurses took their places at my head so I didn't get nervous because the whole world was looking at my lady flower.

Then I got hot.

I got hot and started sweating and couldn't breathe.

The procedure began and—holy shit—*everybody had lied*. No big deal, my *ass!* My entire stomach clamped down, and my insides felt as if they were going to explode. The whole thing lasted only three minutes, and in those three minutes I scanned all of my life experiences up to that point, including all forms of hair waxing as well as high heels. Nothing else ever had the right to cause me pain again. The little tiny tube with the squid ink felt like PVC pipe, and the pressure from the ink being pushed up into my fallopian tubes made me lose my breath, only to catch it long enough to feel as if I might just puke.

As soon as it was over, I sat straight up (and almost passed out) to look at the screen to see if everything was okay. Part of the pain was the panic that my tubes were broken. And before I could express my relief to see that everything was fine as Winnie pointed at my tubes all full of ink, I decided to try to schedule an epidural in advance in case I ever actually experienced labor.

Days later, Dr. New York called us into his office, a fancy one with big windows and a strong wooden desk. "Peanuts?" he asked.

"Sure," I said. "Why not?"

"So, your tubes are clear, as you know, and that's great news. We're starting with a fresh plate." He went on to tell me about the latest research in PCOS and how women were overcoming it with fewer and fewer invasive fertility treatments. "Hardly anyone needs IVF for this."

"What's IVF again?" my husband asked. They use a lot of acronyms in the medical field, and he, understandably, started to lose track.

"In vitro fertilization. It's a catch-all term for getting Erin pregnant by removing her eggs, fertilizing them with your sperm in a petri dish, and then manually implanting them back in her uterus."

"But I don't have to do that, right?" I asked, completely panicked. *IVF is for people who are* really *infertile,* I thought, *not for people like me who are just a* little *infertile and only need to take a few pills and think a couple of good thoughts.*

"I don't think so, Erin. My suggestion is that we begin with a pill to help you ovulate."

See? Just a little pill. Just a little infertile. But I'd read about these pills, and they had side effects. Big side effects. Cramping, exhaustion, nausea, headaches … Even night terrors and psychosis made the list.

"But to be honest," Dr. New York said, "I'm not going to give you one you've heard of or read about before. The latest research suggests we use a pill that is actually given to women who are battling cancer. We aren't completely sure why it works, but it does, and without some of the side effects you've probably read about online."

"Oh, I haven't done *any* reading online, Doctor. I completely trust you." Once my nose grew long enough for him to swat it out of the way, we had a good chuckle and moved along.

"So, if she takes this pill, she'll be able to get pregnant?" Phillip asked.

"The hope is that she will be able to grow viable eggs and get pregnant naturally from there, yes," Dr. New York said.

Phillip and I were quiet.

"'Naturally' meaning the old-fashioned way," Dr. New York clarified.

Phillip and I chuckled because—you know—sex.

I could feel relief flying around between us. We really wanted to do things as naturally as possible so that we could feel a part of the process of creating a son or a daughter.

"I'm going to have a nurse give you a little calendar and some medication. First, you'll need to use a birth control ring for a week to induce your body to have a period. Then you'll follow the instructions and take one of those pills on each of the two days I mark for you on the calendar. After about a week, we'll be able to do an ultrasound to see if the pill worked and your follicles grew. You'll get what we'll call a trigger shot of a hormone to help your eggs move down into your uterus. We can tell you exactly which days to have sex so that your chances are as high as possible. It's all mapped out. You don't have to think."

Yeah, right.

"And, please," Dr. New York added, suddenly more serious, "remember that this is your first fertility cycle. We'll get you pregnant here soon, but be ready. Sometimes women need four or five of these to achieve the results they want."

I nodded. *Of course, of course.* But really. Fertility cycle?

I was not a girl who drank excessively, smoked, or lived an unhealthy lifestyle. I wasn't sick or overweight. I volunteered. I was a good friend. I made birthday gifts instead of buying them so they would feel more personal. I took in abused animals and held funerals for the potted plants I accidentally killed. I came from two parents who drove me around chasing rainbows, for heaven's sake. I was born to be a mother. I knew what kind of parent I would be. I was not someone who *deserved* a fertility disease.

CHAPTER 6

On Not Being Okay

My first fertility cycle included an oral drug and one big fat shot. The pills would make my eggs grow, and if they grew, the big fat shot contained the liquid that would coax my eggs out of my ovaries and into my uterus.

Neither was the sort of medicine you could pick up at your corner pharmacy. This was fancy medication dispensed only from certain pharmacies in certain areas of the country. It felt weird, but also kind of comforting, to know that the method of treatment we were using wasn't available in the grocery store "cough and cold" section.

Several days after my squid ink test, I called a pharmacy in Massachusetts—the Far-Far-Away Pharmacy—and an incredibly helpful woman talked me through the medications listed in the file Dr. New York had already sent to them. She explained what each medicine was for, and, because it's more fun and makes me less liable, I'll make up the names of each one:

"Okay, Erin. I see here we're going to start with a dose of Egg-Growin' Goodness pills. You'll have two of those shipped to you for this twenty-eight-day cycle. Those do not need to be temperature regulated. However, I'm also sending the Giant-Stick-in-Your-Butt Shot liquid on the list, and that needs to be refrigerated. We will send it all directly to your doorstep. Do you have any questions?"

"No. Those are really clearly named medications, so I'm very confident I understand what is happening." Well, I would have said this if those the medications' actual names.

39

The small Styrofoam box landed on my front doorstep two days later. Dr. New York had already given me a birth control ring, which I had I inserted. (It's a magic ring dipped in hormones that you push into your lady business to make you have a period if you need to. Yes, I realize that sounds unrealistic but I'm serious. It's magic.) I cracked open the package and peeked inside. Two pills in a small bottle. Egg-Growin' Goodness, check. One small vial of a clear liquid and one syringe with a four-foot needle. Giant-Stick-in-Your-Butt Shot liquid, check.

Wait. What?

I rushed to the kitchen and pulled everything out of the box and, Mother of God, if there wasn't a needle measuring the length of my arm (that's little to no exaggeration). It was thicker than a soda can. I wondered if this shot was actually going to *phsyically push* the eggs out of my ovaries by force rather than by hormonal trigger.

I stared at the needle. It looked as foreign as it could on my countertop. Then I looked at Charlie and Bella snoring on the living room couch. My first reaction was to go eat a candy bar, but damn it, I couldn't even do that. So I put the needle in the cabinet by the wine glasses along with the two little pills and ignored it, even though it whispered my name and taunted me every time I walked by. ("Errriiin! I'm goonnna stick yooou!")

One week after I got my period thanks to the magic ring, I took the first little Egg-Growin' Goodness pill. It was about the size of a Tic Tac. It looked like a Tic Tac too. In hindsight, I was possible that I had just spent several hundred dollars on Tic Tacs, but regardless of whether they were real medication or one big placebo, I was going to find out if my eggs grew. I took the second pill the next day and then scheduled my next appointment for an ultrasound, during which the nurses would measure the size of my follicles.

Remember follicles? They are little sacs in my ovaries that release my eggs. We want big follicles because that means the eggs inside are ready to become babies.

My first ultrasound was in the New Orleans room at Dr. New York's office. I climbed up onto the table and waited with my peanuts. Phillip read something on his phone. We were both super nervous until Winnie bounced in.

Winnie was on the short side and had curly hair—the hair I stared at longingly until she'd caused me more pain than three stubbed toes and a paper cut during the HSG test she'd administered a few weeks before. Her midlife face was all knowing, but her wrinkles only stayed wrinkly near the parts of her face that laughed.

"Good mooo-ooorning!" Winnie sang. "Today's the day we measure your big, fat follicles! You know, Erin, it is so smart that you always wear skirts and dresses to these appointments. Just so smart."

She turned on the machine, and I hiked up my skirt so she could begin the procedure. You see, ultrasounds aren't like you see on TV unless you're well into a pregnancy. They don't cover your belly in jelly and rub the X-ray vision camera back and forth to see your insides on a big screen. No, these are *internal* ultrasounds. Lie back, ladies, and put your feet up in the stirrups so your flight attendant can insert a slightly uncomfortable, slick, long X-ray vision camera into your vagina and then angle it at your ovaries to see what there is to see on the big screen. Want a cocktail? You can't have one because you can't have sugar, so here, enjoy this water and a stick of sugar-free gum.

I would need to do this two or three times per fertility cycle, plus once a week if I got pregnant until I was ten weeks pregnant. So, if I got pregnant within the average five months most girls do, I would have upwards of thirty internal ultrasounds. *Thirty.*

Winnie used the mouse pad attached to the machine to measure circles on the screen, and she wrote down numbers as she moved the camera around. The silence was palpable as I searched the screen, trying to figure out what I was looking at. I hoped and prayed that I would be one of the girls that Pam, the other nurse, had told me about—the girls who responded to the first round of fertility drugs, grew awesome eggs, and got pregnant right away.

"Oooo-kay!" Winnie said brightly. "This is oooo-kay!"

I could tell immediately by the tone of her voice that we hadn't made progress. She was being faux perky, trying to keep me upbeat. No visible wrinkles near her eyes. I returned the effort with a smile, trying to be oooo-kay with the fact that my follicles clearly hadn't grown, but I couldn't make eye contact with Phil for fear my eyes would well up.

Had I eaten sugar accidentally? Had I not been positive enough? I wasn't exercising, but maybe I was walking too much? Was I going to be doing this for years? I flashed forward to a lifetime of fertility treatments, as if this was just the beginning of hundreds of experiences just like this one. Thousands of internal ultrasounds.

Then I started to feel hot shame. I had gotten us into this mess. I was the one with the body that didn't work. I was the one who was signing us up for medications flown in from Massachusetts and ultrasounds that cost a few hundred dollars a pop.

I do this. I take what's happening right now and I turn it into forever. *I will always be infertile. I will never have a child.* Whether it's my favorite sushi restaurant closing or my father dying, I drop hope the second life gets hard. Hope hurts. Hope is way too vulnerable for me. If I have no hope, then at least I get a nice surprise every now and again. But with this feeling of forever shooting through my heart, it rarely ever occurred to me that what I want might not be as good as what's coming, and that hope could be worth it. I desperately wanted to give up in that moment. I wanted to rip the stupid ultrasound wand out of my vagina and walk straight to the car and say forget it. But for the first time in my life, I wanted something more than I wanted to feel okay.

For the first time in my life, I was going to find out if I could survive not being okay.

I got a hold of myself in the stirrups and refocused. *Okay, Erin. It's the first try. You're working and so is Phillip, and we can afford this. There are many options. There are many possibilities. Don't give up yet.*

"What do we do next?" I asked Winnie with a deep breath.

She smiled with compassion. Then she said firmly, "We try again."

Okay, I thought. *That's okay. We're just going to try again, and next time will be better. Until ….*

"Winnie," I said, "I ordered the Giant-Stick-in-Your-Butt Shot that I'm supposed to get when my follicles grow. If my follicles don't grow, what do I do with the Giant-Stick-in-Your-Butt Shot?"

Winnie explained I should keep that Giant-Stick-in-Your-Butt Shot at home (that big needle chuckled when she said that) and just wait a few days because *maybe* my follicles were late bloomers. "That happens sometimes! Small follicles on Monday then—*wow!*—big follicles on

Wednesday!" There was still a chance this cycle could be the one that gave us a pregnancy. There was still a chance.

I went home and did the only thing I knew to do to get my follicles to grow. I started each morning by putting my hands over my tummy and singing, "Grow, follicles! Grow! Yooou can dooo it!" Phillip occasionally sang backup. "Grow, grow!"

If I felt a funny feeling in my tummy, I focused on it and willed it to be the right feeling, and then I distracted myself with *not sugar*. I listened to audio books, I worked, I cleaned, I organized. I never let myself go past an initial pang of anxiety for fear that letting it all go would kill me.

Two days later, Winnie greeted me with a smile in the Kauai room for my next appointment. My friends had honeymooned in Kauai. Was *that* a sign?

"You ready for some follicles, girl?" Winnie exclaimed.

I was, but I had a gut feeling (no pun intended) that nothing else had happened. And as it turned out, my guts have a pretty high IQ. Nothing. The follicles were still small. Nobody grew, not even one. We'd have to scrap the entire cycle.

Now, here's the thing about failing at fertility. It's not as though you can pick up and try again where you left off. You have to wait. You have to let your body reboot with the magic birth control ring and then proceed with the next round of pills and waiting. It's not like normal life equations where there's a cause and then an immediately reaction. There's a setup involved in this life equation. A pre-equation equation. I couldn't think of the outcome of the equation because I had no idea if the setup would even lead to the equation, let alone the outcome. I knew right then I was going to have to live my life in three-week chunks and never think past that. Life would be in limbo until (and if) we got pregnant. I started to focus only on two- or three-week chunks, and eventually focused only on the day I was in. It became a hard and fast rule for survival.

"Do you want to go to dinner tomorrow night with Howard and Ashley?" Phillip asked. It was a Thursday, and I was cleaning the kitchen, wiping down counters and pointedly (get it?) ignoring the cabinet that was housing the Giant-Stick-in-Your-Butt Shot.

I glanced over at him. "I don't know. It's not tomorrow night yet."

"Okay, well ..." He glanced down at his phone, receiving a text. "They're going to a hibachi grill. Do you think you can eat anything there?"

"Um, I can't eat rice. Or anything fried. I could eat the chicken and the vegetables, but none of the sauces. And I couldn't drink sake. I could just bring something and sit with you all."

Phillip was quiet for a moment. "I think they're going around eight, so I'll just let them know we'll try to make it."

"Fine," I said, feeling defensive and prickly. "But I'm not making any promises. Plus, eight is late. I need to get to bed to ensure I'm getting enough rest. I probably shouldn't go. You can go."

And that was how planning went.

I wanted the whole world to stop asking me about tomorrow or next month. I wanted my husband to stand at the front door and turn away all of the people who might have a question about anything further in the future than *today*. I wanted him to announce, "We shall not be thinking of the future in this house until further notice. If you want to know about the future, you'll just have to wait."

More specifically, I wanted him to tell people we could go to dinner and then wait until the *day* of the dinner to actually tell me about it.

I wanted Phillip to protect me from the future and everything scary that could happen there and just live with me, right there in every single moment, like my mom used to do. I had absolutely no proof that I could survive disappointment.

But that was hard to articulate then. I'm not sure if it bothered Phillip that I could only live in today; he never really acknowledged it. And even though I was living day to day, I still wasn't *present*. I was numb. Just numb enough, floating in the perfect amount of self-induced anesthesia to stay functional. A little to the left, and I would have been on the couch unable to move. A little to the right, and I would be in manic panic, questioning the outcome of every possible scenario we might face.

Infertility can do weird things to a marriage. It can cause you to grow closer or it can cause you to blame each other. What's weirder is that it didn't really do either of those things to our marriage. Neither of us talked about the infertility, but we didn't avoid the subject either. We didn't fight about it. We didn't cry about it (together). All of our friends knew what was going on, but it wasn't dinner conversation. Infertility became a way of life, a roommate. Phillip passed the starchy potatoes over my head as they went around the big family dinner table, and I reminded him when our appointments were (and he showed up for every one of them), and that was how we lived.

Neutral.

There were days I wanted to scream at him, "Do you even want to have a baby with me?" I wanted so much to ask him if he was scared or if he ever thought about adoption if this didn't work. But I didn't want to seem "crazy" or hormonal. I'm not even sure I wanted to know what he'd say in any of these scenarios because I was afraid I might not be able to handle it. I was downright scared. Was he?

Instead of sharing any of that with him, I kept a calendar of our appointments and a list of the foods I could eat on the kitchen counter and put one foot in front of the other. I wouldn't suggest that. As painful as sharing the sharp pangs of infertility with your partner can be, you're the only two people who can relate to the situation. No one else understands it the way you two do. I wish I had shared more, asked more questions, and allowed my fear to be seen. In hindsight, I understand that holding it in was so much harder.

At our next appointment, Winnie (who had performed that squid ink test the week before and told me that my follicles hadn't seemed to grow) met us back in the Kaui room for one final ultrasound to officially label this cycle a dud. I prayed on the table, feet in the stirrups, that maybe I had those unicorn follicles that surprised everyone by growing at the last minute.

I didn't.

"Welp, just as we suspected." She smiled at the screen and not me. "It's okay. We're going again!" Winnie told us that it was time to add injectable fertility drugs into the beginning of each cycle to try to get things rolling.

I was in no way ready to hear that.

After I had a mild panic attack, Winnie told me how much the injectable drugs cost. This took me from panic attack to seizure. I'm pretty sure the Care Bears and the Smurfs walked in right after she said the number and started fighting and sticking each other with needles, screaming, "Ahhh! We're going to make babies! Everything's gone wrong! Ahhhh!"

My husband's immediate reaction was, "All right, let's do it."

I shook my head no.

With every step we were taking to try to make a baby, I became less and less a female and felt more and more that I was in the middle of a game of Battleship. Do I hang out and let them continue poking me until they sink the whole ship?

Phillip looked at me trying to understand the magnificent feeling of loss I was expressing with a single word. But he couldn't really. After all, the point of being a woman is to have the babies. Thinking I was unable to have babies myself was creating a fracture between who I always thought I was meant to be and who it actually turned out that I was.

This experience cannot be the same for a man; it simply can't. As unfair as it seems when a child is born, that child is not yet a part of the man (aside from his very important DNA). It is *very* much a part of the woman, a piece from inside now moved outside. It's *our* job to grow, birth, and feed our children. If I couldn't even do that, who was I? What was my purpose? I mean, all I did was get a blood test to find out if maybe something was wrong and now, a few months later, I was listening to a nurse suggest injectable fertility medication. How had this even happened?

"It'll happen!" Winnie rubbed my shin from where she stood at the bottom of the exam table. "I've seen three girls today—boom, boom, boom! All three pregnant. We'll get there!"

Awesome, I thought. Three girls, all pregnant. So that made me the barren twenty-eight-year-old with no hope of ever fulfilling my biological purpose here on Earth. "Were those girls' symptoms as bad as mine?" I wanted to ask. "How many months did it take them to get pregnant? Did they take cinnamon supplements?"

I was sent to the Telluride room to wait for a nurse to talk to me about our options. It had been almost two months since I'd been diagnosed with PCOS. Two months passes in the blink of an eye when you're not trying to get pregnant, but it felt like twenty years since the night Phillip and I had looked at each other in the car and said, "So we're trying?"

I cried a few tears and as Winnie passed by Telluride. She saw me and paused in the doorway. "It's fine. We'll get you there. It's fine."

"It's not fine!" I snapped. "It's my only job! I'm the girl, and I make the babies! And I can't do my job if my follicles won't grow. I'm going to become a pin cushion, not a mother." Having watched hundreds of girls before me experience this same feeling, Winnie knew the best thing she could do was sit down and silently put her arm around me.

This was perhaps the four hundredth thousandth time I'd said this over the course of this experience, but I meant it every time.

Pam came in next and saw tears in my eyes. She put her hand on my back and said, "No! Don't cry! We just have to find the recipe, sweetie. The perfect pregnancy recipe for you. We will find it, and I promise, we will get you pregnant."

"Promise?" I asked, like a crying five-year-old.

"Promise." Pam smiled.

• • • • • • • • • • • • • • • • • • •

I spent the next two weeks at Target, which most women will tell you can cure even the worst depression. You probably never knew you needed *that* many picture frames.

One night, after my evening Target run, Phillip and I sat down to do the finances. We realized that, after all the medical bills piled up we were starting to accumulate credit card debt, something we'd never had. Even if we began paying off next month's medical bills in full, injectables included, we wouldn't have any money left over to pay the minimum on the credit cards! So *this* was how America had gotten into the worst economic situation of our time: fertility drugs!

We put a spending freeze on all credit cards and broke down to the bare essentials every month, including food, electricity, gas, and mortgage. We ate out only once a week (with a coupon from the circular) and never bought breakfast or lunch out. I stopped buying things for the dogs, I used coupons and followed the sales, and (dun, dun, dun!) I stopped going to Target. This, as it turns out, was how I would come to define a mother's ultimate sacrifice.

We'd decided to move forward with the injectables, mainly because Winnie's last words to me on the way out of the office were, "Oh, take the next step, honey. You want to have a baby? Have a baby. You won't even remember everything you went through once that little joy is here. Just do it!"

That night, I called the Far-Far-Away Pharmacy and asked if they had my prescription on file.

"Hi, Ms. Salem! I have your prescription right here! And you also qualify for our medical assistance program."

"Huh? I didn't sign up for that."

"Oh, you don't have to. We automatically apply it to all accounts with Dr. New York."

"Why?" I asked. "Is the total that high?"

"Well, you are ordering the injectables today. Those cost—"

"*Wait!*" I interrupted. "I don't want to know."

"You don't want to know the price?"

"Nope."

"Okay. Well, I can just give you the total of the order so you know what we're charging you."

"Nope. Don't want to know that either."

She paused. She was clearly surprised. This wasn't one of the options in her script. "Okay, Ms. Salem, well, we'll be charging your credit card a total of … um … we'll just be charging it. And if you have any questions about the cost, then you can … um … you can call us."

"Sounds great!" I hung up, called my husband, and told him I would not be looking at the credit card bill this month.

It ain't just a river in Egypt.

I later learned that the injectable medication alone was nearly $1,500 a month. Along with the ultrasounds, we were spending every penny I earned on infertility treatments. On one hand, I felt blessed to have a job to pay these bills. On the other hand, I felt deep resentment that most women spent nothing (except for maybe a $15 pregnancy test).

• • • • • • • • • • • • • • • • • • •

I was writing in my journal everyday about "feelings" and "dreams." I wrote so much that I started to lose the focus of my life. Everyday became a big pity party.

Waaah, we have no money.

Waaah, I can't eat cookies.

Waaah, I'm infertile.

Other than my mom, Phillip, and his sister Sharon I didn't talk to many people about what we were going through. Frankly, no one knew what to say. It's hard to know how to help someone having fertility treatments. People don't want to ask about it, but they also want to talk about it and find out what's going on. They forget it's your body—your physical being—that isn't working, not a washing machine that you can eventually fix or replace after it causes all kinds of nuisance with dirty laundry.

I had several girlfriends who weren't pregnant but who tried relating to me. "Yeah, I felt that way when we were trying to close on our house." And as valiant as it was that they tried to relate to me, *No, you didn't feel this way when you were trying to close on your house. You didn't feel anything close to this.*

If I had it to do again, I would have asked more people to listen. Just listen. I would have cried more to Phillip or found a support group (online or in person). I would have dropped the concern of annoying someone I trusted with my fear and pain and truly let them see me. Retreating into myself made an already difficult process harder.

Loneliness is hard to recognize when you're feeling it, and I was so focused on getting pregnant that I didn't realize how alone I felt. I filled the space in dubious ways: I read abundant amounts of information about infertility in Google Doctor School. I watched endless hours of TV shows about parenting, babies, and birth. Oh, the birth shows. I watched those a lot. I pushed with those women every day at two and then again at two thirty. Eventually, I did fall far enough to the left that I got pretty depressed. I got so depressed that I couldn't enjoy much of anything. My every thought was consumed with babies and fertility and beating this battle. People started to worry about me. Even I started to worry about me.

Then, one day, I read an article about joy and how it could affect your health. Purposeful joy can actually change our brains! My depressed mind said, "That's crap!" But a little birdie deep in my soul said, "That could be a key to all of this. Maybe a life lesson, even. Chirp. Chirp."

CHAPTER 7

Interceptions and Injectables

When I was seven years old and sat in the hospital break room in the hours following my father's death, everyone told me I was strong and brave. Brave and strong, that's me. And when you're seven, you believe people who tell you that, not because it's what you are but because it's what you assume you have to be in order to survive. I thought I needed to keep it all together so no one—especially my mother, still falling apart in the next room—had to worry about me. I should be strong and brave. Now, as a fatherless twenty-eight-year old, seeking joy seemed like a new version of being strong and brave.

After reading the joy article, I was determined to change the trajectory. Eight years earlier, on the day that two airplanes flew into the Twin Towers in New York City while I was in a theatre management class, I had spiraled all the way down. I ended up on antidepressants and antianxiety medications for a year, plus another medication to help me sleep. Now, I had absolutely no idea how to keep myself from sinking lower and lower into my fear and depression again without those medications. My doctor recommended I not go back on antidepressants while taking all these infertility drugs because they could potentially make it more difficult to get pregnant. I was forced to make some changes that would—hopefully—keep me from spiraling down again.

So, I stopped writing sad feelings in my journal. Instead, I wrote about a few things I was glad about each day. (A lot of times, I was "glad I like nuts," or "glad grass grows," or "glad I have a toilet." But at least it was something to be glad about.) I dropped out of the Google Medical School (much to my mother's dismay, but at least I still had Google Law School).

I quit reading books related to pregnancy, and I stopped watching other women have babies on TV. Instead, I made a game out of cooking on the cheap and reusing old clothes to make new outfits. I planned fun and free things to do with my husband and dogs. I watched only football games and funny movies. I even got jokey with the people who asked me questions or tried to comfort me about my situation, and often times in ended up in a good laugh instead of a sad, "I'm so sorry this is happening to you." I got so wrapped up enjoying life without fertility-cycle-on-the-brain, I almost forgot I was infertile! What joy!

Okay, so the joy wasn't *quite* real. It was fake joy. It was mostly an act. But I figured acting joyful was better than actually *being* depressed. Besides, it was working.

The real joy—and about the only joy—came from writing my blog. I had started a blog before we left LA to keep friends and family on the West Coast up to date with our travels and new life in Florida. But as the time went on, I began to realize how much I enjoyed writing about my real thoughts, feelings, and experiences unrelated to the move. But telling a funny anecdote about painting the living room suddenly felt dishonest, as if I was intentionally hiding this huge thing happening in our lives. There were bigger things I wanted to say.

So I decided to write about my fertility treatments. I thought maybe I would lose readers—those people who came to the blog for a quick funny story, an easy laugh. Instead, women gravitated toward the *real* me. The *honest* me. They cared about what I was going through and, even more amazing, they shared with me what *they* were going through.

Many of them had experienced PCOS. Lots had dealt with endometriosis, fibroids, miscarriages, or in my opinion the very worst—unexplained infertility. And because the internet was lush with websites talking about symptoms and treatments, but actually very little about the emotional side of infertility, women wrote to me every day asking me questions. No one expected me to be an expert. They just wanted to know that someone else was experiencing this frustration with them.

When they did ask me specific questions about my PCOS, I was able to share so much about my experience: the treatments I was trying, how I was diagnosed, what I understood about the way the syndrome manifested in me. Some women knew a lot more than I did and gave me advice; and some felt as if their doctors hadn't explained nearly as much as mine had, so they felt armed with information after our exchanges.

Dear Erin,

I've been reading your blog. No one in my family knows we're struggling with infertility. I have polyps in my uterus that we just had removed earlier this year. Now I'm being asked to take the drug Clomid. Have you ever taken that one?

Knowing that someone else is going through this makes me feel less alone. I just want you to know it's helping me. Keep writing.

Sincerely,

Polly

Dear Polly,

I'm so sorry you're going through it too. Sometimes it helps to talk to strangers instead of family, right?

Was the polyp removal painful?

I never took Clomid because my doctor said it wasn't the right drug for me. But he did mention it as being one he often prescribes. You'll have to tell me how it goes.

We're in this together, Polly. Keep reading.

Love,

Erin

It felt good to be a source of awareness and even answer questions for some women. It gave me a meaningful sense of purpose, something I'd been searching for since our move almost ten months earlier. In three hundred words a day or less, I found purpose. And that purpose brought me the joy I needed to push through the next round of treatment.

Actual joy.

It was fleeting, but it was real.

• • • • • • • • • • • • • • • • • • • •

The next ultrasound visit came a week after I took the Egg-Growin' Goodness pills again. The nurses all said hi and asked about my life as I walked through the halls to my ultrasound room.

"Hey, girl!" Winnie would say. "How are your dogs?!"

"Whatcha makin' for dinner tonight, Erin?" Pam would ask.

I almost felt as if we were all friends who met up once a week to look at each other's ovaries, except I never saw theirs (story of my life). This made for fairly weird friendships, but friendships nonetheless.

I sat up on the table waiting for Winnie or Pam to come in and see me. My husband sat next to me in a chair reading a pregnancy magazine. I watched him turn pages, wondering if he could possibly be as absorbed as he seemed as he studied the story about a woman who gave birth in her back yard. When the door opened, my cheery smile froze a little: it was Dr. New York who walked in.

Let me clarify: Dr. New York was *a man*. A *man* who wanted to give me an internal ultrasound. (Remember those?) While I trusted him implicitly and loved his bedside manner, I'd never ever had a man examine my flower before.

I got flushed and flustered. I automatically started talking about football, hoping we could relate and find common ground before he started "working."

"Hey, Doc!" I said, way too brightly. "Who's your college team?"

"Oh, yeah, I'm not much of a college ball guy. I like the Jags."

"Yes! Oh sure. Me, too. I mean, they're not my team. I'm a Steelers fan. Did you see that game on Sunday?"

"I didn't. I didn't see it. We were moving this past weekend, and ..." He sat on a small stool with wheels and maneuvered in front of me. He motioned for me to lie back and put my feet in the stirrups. I did so but started talking faster and asking more questions.

"Oh!" I exclaimed. "It was unbelievable! Do you like going to the games? Can you believe they let you take food in now? Do you have season tickets? What food do you like?"

I didn't listen to any of his responses. I just watched his hands as they stretched the gloves and reached toward the ultrasound machine to pick up the wand and press buttons. Thankfully, my husband continued the football-related fodder while I reclined, stunned. Winnie popped her head in and smiled. I craned my neck to look at her, sending her telepathic messages: *Code Blue! A man is in this room attempting to do my internal ultrasound. A* man!

Winnie did not understand the fundamentals of telepathy. She just waved hello bigger and walked out. So I held my breath and hoped I could focus on his questions without crying and yelling, "You're a man!"

It all went away when I saw the screen.

The pills had worked this time.

The Egg-Growin' Goodness pills had grown eggs. Well, follicles. I could see right there, right in front of me, that the follicles were twice the size they had been the previous month. Dr. New York measured them on the screen, drawing lines with the arrows and noting measurements on the keyboard. And there was more than one!

"Great!" Dr. New York the Man said. "These look great! Viable! We can go ahead and start the injectables! I just hope you don't have too many follicles grow because you are responding so well!"

You hear that? *Overachiever!*

"We don't want you to be the next mother of nine babies," he continued, "so we'll keep a close eye on everything, but so far this is great."

Hahaha! We all laughed and slapped our knees. Oh, Dr. New York the Man! Ohhh, what a hoot. What a gay old time we were having! Progress and jokes. Could this day get better?

Dr. New York opened the door a crack and said, "Pam, will you please have Sally take them into the other room to teach them how to do the injections."

What?

"What?" I cried. "Who does the injections?"

"You do!" Dr. New York the Man said with an easy smile, as if we were still sharing a funny. "Or your husband, if that makes you more comfortable."

Husband sticking me with needles: comfortable fail.

"You'll be fine. Sally will teach you!" Dr. New York the Man smiled, high-fived my husband, and then left the room.

I pulled my skirt down in silence and put on my shoes until Phillip finally said, "It'll be fine. They wouldn't let me do the shots if it wasn't routine. I'm sure plenty of people have done it themselves before."

I tried to keep my composure. Instead of saying, "Um, *doctors* give shots. In a *doctor's* office. With a sterile environment and years of medical practice. You have a theatre degree and work in commercial real estate. You aren't qualified to give me shots in our kitchen next to the *coffee pot*." What I really said was, "Yeah. I'm sure you're right."

Pam met us in the hall and told us to head over to the Lake Como room to meet Sally the Shot Nurse.

Sally the Shot Nurse often greeted us as we arrived or helped us get to our next vacation-named exam room, but she'd never seen my cervix before, so as far as I was concerned, she was a complete stranger. She was tall, with dark wavy hair and a quiet demeanor. She moved fluidly, comfortable in her own skin. She let out a sweet "Hellooo!" and whipped out a needle and some little glass jars. I stopped breathing. She revived me. The demonstration continued.

She explained that the vials of liquid at home making up the team of The Injectables would continue to encourage the follicles to grow in case they considered stalling out like they had last time. She showed us how to put the right needle on the top of the plunger, suck the liquid into the syringe, and then puncture my stomach. She used a fake little tummy about the size of an apple to demonstrate. When she was finished, I asked her if she could do the entire demonstration again. She laughed.

"I'm not kidding," I said.

She paused before Phillip smiled and shook his head. "We'll be fine," he said, much more reassuringly than he had the right to be.

"Be right back," she said.

Sally the Shot Nurse left the room and came back with an informational DVD. "No one ever actually watches this," she said with a giggle, "but you can take it home if you want."

I took the DVD from her hands. I'd watch it eighty-seven times if it meant we'd do this right. "Thank you," I said, slipping it into my bag.

"You'll take these three shots at night between the hours of six and nine, okay?" Sally asked.

"No problem!" I said.

This was no problem.

Except for the fact that there was one problem.

Phillip's parents had bought us tickets to the Florida/Georgia game on the second night of The Injectables. For those of you who don't currently or have never lived in Florida, good for you. Also, you should know these are the nights we live for. College football nights, *especially* Florida/Georgia when you're allowed to scream and drink and act like idiots over the colors of a school you probably didn't even attend. It's an all-day event. Tailgating starts early in the morning, and by the time you get to the game, you're so incredibly pumped up that it doesn't matter if they end up playing a giant game of tiddlywinks—you just want to *win!*

"Oh, just go to the bathroom at the stadium and do it!" Sally the Shot Nurse said when I ran back to her from the front desk.

Now, getting an injection in my kitchen was a terrible idea. It was where we cut raw meat and spilled sticky sauces. But I could live with it. Getting an injection in the bathroom at a Florida game was unconscionable. That was where twenty-year-old college students spent the second quarter puking their brains out on the floor because they couldn't make it to the toilet and then got wheeled out by a security guard while their peers followed, shouting, "One more drink! One more drink!" Not to mention there was poo in there.

So I was left with a choice: convince my husband to leave the Florida game early or face certain death in a stadium bathroom. When I weighed out the risk/reward factors of both, I decided to adopt.

The first day of The Injectables brought massive anticipation. I tried pretending nothing was going to happen that evening. Maybe I would be cooking and—bloop!—my husband would stab me in the stomach, and I would serve dinner! Maybe I would be almost asleep on the couch and—hey-o!—my husband would insert a needle into my stomach, and I'd go right off to dreamland.

When he got home from work, Phillip stood tall and casual in demeanor. He hovered over our kitchen counter, carefully mixing and combining the liquids while I stirred a lovely chicken sauce on the stove. His dark brown eyes studied the bottles as he followed the instructions from Sally the Shot Nurse. He speaks aloud when he's doing most anything, which used to drive me crazy: "And then the popcorn kernels go in the pot." "Next I grab the screwdriver." "Now I'll need—let's see—three more feet of …"

As soon as I heard him say, "Screw the needle on the plunger." I grabbed an ice cube from the freezer and held it on my belly in the spot where he would stab me. I stood, stirring and icing, occasionally glancing down at the reddening patch of skin and waiting for the panic attack to set in.

And then, Phillip turned around with a syringe bearing the longest needle I'd ever seen. I gasped and shouted, "That's not the right needle!"

He responded calmly. "Yes, it is, sweetie. It's the same needle the nurse showed us in the office."

Mind you, Sally the Shot Nurse had clearly stated that the needle should be plunged *in its entirety* into my stomach. If that needle went all the way into my stomach, my husband would inject hormones directly into my uterus. It was *that* long. I started hyperventilating. *This can't be right! You cannot give a man permission to stab his wife with a needle that long!* I dropped the ice cube and started rummaging through the boxes on my kitchen counter. I pulled out bags of extra syringes and little glass jars in multiple sizes. I frantically looked through every baggie and small box, praying that the needle in my husband's hands was the wrong needle.

And guess what?

It was the wrong needle.

He hadn't even *read* the baggie he took the needle from, and the baggie happened to be for the Giant-Stick-in-Your-Butt Shot that I wasn't supposed to get for another week, not The Injectables! Phillip was about to skewer me like so much teriyaki beef on the Giant-Stick-in-Your-Butt Shot! See? This is why husbands should never be allowed to give their wives shots in the kitchen!

"You were about to stab me with Giant-Stick-in-Your-Butt Shot needle!" I yelled. "This is not the right needle! Are you ever paying attention? Did you watch the DVD? This is important! You were going to stab me in the stomach with that! You could have killed me!"

I was a little upset.

And not just about nearly becoming a human kabob, but because of what this little mistake might have cost us. There was currently $160 of liquid floating in a little syringe with the wrong needle on top. How the hell were we going to get the liquid into the right syringe with the right needle? Was it possible to transport the liquid out of the wrong needle, through the right needle, and down into a new syringe? Could we siphon it out with a bendy straw? Was I supposed run to the hospital with the syringe in hand and scream, "My husband isn't a doctor and tried to be one in my kitchen!"?

What should someone do in this situation?

While I panicked, Phillip stayed very calm. He held the syringe in one hand while sifting through the pile of needles on the counter. He picked up the right needle and looked at it carefully, light glinting off his glasses. And in a moment of brilliance, he carefully unscrewed the Giant-Stick-in-Your-Butt Shot needle from the syringe and replaced it with a smaller needle—without losing a drop of fertility goodness. Syringes now come with screw top needles. Finally, the medical world is taking cues from the wine world.

When the correct needle was in place, I leaned back against the counter and closed my eyes. My heart was still pounding, and I was so hot that the little spot I'd numbed on my belly was right back to feeling like a little spot.

"Are you ready?" Phillip asked, carefully watching my face.

"Yes, just do it."

He squeezed a little hunk of flesh on my belly. "Deep breath."

"Just do it!"

He took a short breath and started to count. Counting was the last thing I wanted him to do at this moment. But it was happening, and before I could shout, "Stop counting!" my brain interrupted with the thought that Phillip could drop the syringe if I screamed or he could accidentally stab me straight through the belly button and *then* where would we be?!

Boink!

In all that thinking, it was over. I was red and sweaty and breathing really fast, but it was over. We had just successfully completed our first injectable. We both took a deep breath.

"You were so calm," I told him, looking at him with fresh admiration.

"Well, of course, babe," Phillip said, setting the syringe aside. "You needed me to be calm. I'm here for you."

I smiled and sank back against the kitchen counter, staring at the injection site on my belly. I quietly rejoiced in how lucky I was to have a man who knew how to deal with stressful situations. Never once did Phillip lose his cool or allow my stress levels to make him nervous. I was truly blessed.

Then, with a shit-I-need-a-drink laugh, Phillip said, "Man! I am so glad that's over. That was really scary, huh? I almost peed my pants!"

• • • • • • • • • • • • • • • • • • • •

The morning of the Florida game (injectable day two), I packed my syringes and little glass jars in a lunch box that I used to take to work with me. I couldn't let The Injectables get too hot or their superpowers would be squelched. I had to pack ice around the jars so they didn't get too warm. I also packed sugar-free cookies. You know, typical game day supplies: syringes and cookies.

Though Sally the Shot Nurse had said Phillip could administer a shot in a stadium bathroom if need be, I desperately wanted to avoid that fate.

We drove to the game with his parents and spent an afternoon baking in the sun with Phillip's family. I kept checking to make sure my lunch box was safe in the car and that the ice hadn't melted. I checked it so many times you'd think it *was* a baby. I also thought about it the entire time I was inside the game. *I wonder if the lunchbox feels lonely? I wonder if it's too hot or too cold? I wonder if it knows I'm coming back for it?*

It was normal for my husband's family to leave a Florida game early if it was clear our team would win. This happened more often than not. So at about seven in the evening, when our team was *clearly* winning, I asked Phillip if we could leave early. He looked at his mom and asked, "Can we leave early?"

I gave her the *Shrek* Puss in Boots big eyes.

She said to Phillip, "Ask your father."

We all turned our heads in a big, waving motions toward my father-in-law, who said, "Oh, I'd like to stay."

Now, this man rarely expressed an opinion. He was happy to go with the flow of his family. So when he said he wanted to stay, we stayed. Damn it, we stayed.

Damn it.

I stared at my watch until seven thirty when the game finally ended. I knew we could do the shots at home (where I wanted to do them) if we could just make it there by nine. There was just one problem: the entire city was parked in the stadium parking lot. By the time we got to the car it would be eight. I envisioned us in the back seat of Phillip's parents' van trying to hold syringes and vials steady over the potholes and sudden stops to avoid hitting drunk Florida fans.

Then my phone rang, and I saw that it was a dear old friend, Darlene. She and I had met in sixth grade and had become instant friends. We spent our high school years being theatre nerds, practicing musical numbers for no one and watching episodes of very bad daytime talk shows ad nauseam. We learned to drive together, started dating boys together, and experienced the ups and downs of life together until we were eighteen. And while we didn't talk as much as we wanted to anymore, our love never wavered. I picked up for a nice distraction.

"Where have you been?" she burst out.

"I was at the Florida game all day! Sorry!"

"I've been trying to call you!"

"Oh! I didn't mean to worry you. Everything okay?"

She sighed. "Yes. Everything okay with you? Pregnant yet?"

"No, I'm not pregnant. Other than that, I'm fine."

"Sorry, babe," she said. She always asked if I was pregnant. She always lamented with me when I wasn't. It was nice to have a teammate.

"So what's new with you?" I asked while Phillip's parent's drove off the interstate. Almost home.

"Well, I was calling you all day to tell you—" I immediately started screaming. I knew exactly what she was about to say, and I couldn't get any words out except for the highest-pitched scream ever. I broke glass. Dogs came running from everywhere. Dolphins held their ears with their fins.

My friend was pregnant.

I completely lost track of how important the shots were and, once we got home, wandered around the house talking to her about how she was feeling and how thrilled I was for her. We always said we would be pregnant together, and I never expected it could actually happen. And here she was, pregnant and waiting for me to hurry up and meet her there.

Phillip was ready to give me the shot. I had so much adrenaline rushing through my veins while I was on that phone call that he just went ahead and poked me while I talked, and the shot didn't even hurt. In fact, it felt good. I was one step closer to being pregnant with my friend this month!

CHAPTER 8

Pasta and Orgasms—My Long-Lost Friends

The Injectables shots became as easy as peeling a hard-boiled egg and pairing it with bacon every single morning for the rest of my life. In fact, my husband administered the third shot while I was lying in bed watching TV and he was drinking a gluten-free beer. I don't recommend this; neither do I support my own decision to publish that last line, but it's for the best that you know all the facts.

It was around that third shot that I began to feel tired and lumpy. I wasn't getting much exercise because, according to Dr. New York, cardio would release the "wrong hormones."

As a result of my new sedentary lifestyle, my body was no longer lean and mean. It was kind of soft and apathetic instead. My butt, which three months earlier had been a taut and stand-up gal, had just kind of laid down for a nap. My arms had previously sported a hot little line that shouted "Check me out! I'm muscles!" Now, without the line, they resembled small, droopy flags waving even when I wasn't. The skin used to stretch tightly over my well-defined thighs and calves, but no more. And my stomach? Oh, my stomach. I'm not sure I even want to say something witty about it.

I started to think that my food might be making me depressed—not physiologically, but emotionally. I missed pasta. The unbelievable joy of a heaping plate of spaghetti topped with my mama's marinara makes my heart beat faster and my mouth water right this minute. I would have kissed a snake enveloped in a mass of spiders for a huge bowl of oatmeal with strawberries in the morning or a piece of peanut butter toast. And the connection my husband and I used to make over an incredible date-night meal had been missing from our lives. Sure, Phillip and I could connect over a perfectly sugar-free, starch-free meal, but it usually sounded something like:

"I miss pasta."

"Yeah. Me too."

There was just something about good food—real food, food that reminded us of our childhoods or favorite vacations. It was a common denominator. Every major milestone in our relationship we could relate to food. Our first date, we marinated and cooked a venison tenderloin. We were twenty. When Phil visited me after college, I would make him a huge pot of my mama's sauce with gorgeous, long strands of spaghetti drooping off the plate. The meal we ate in LA when we knew we would get married (but didn't say it) included rabbit, short ribs, and the most glorious scallops ever created, all served with fresh, crunchy bread. We knew how to eat, and we loved sharing in the experience. Never-ending salads with grilled chicken were exhausting us both.

Despite desperately missing the food I loved to cook and eat, I didn't change anything. When Dr. New York told me this diet would get me pregnant, I felt tied to it. Deviating even just a little meant that a negative pregnancy test could be my fault.

Growing up a theatre rat, I knew the difference between being turned down for a role because I was unprepared and being turned down for a role because I wasn't right for it. I applied the same logic here. Even one small bite of ice cream or one short cardio burst in the middle of a casual walk—that's all I would be able to think about if I were to stare at the minus sign of a pregnancy test. But if I stuck to the diet and the rules to a T and I wasn't pregnant, well, I knew it couldn't be my fault.

My ultrasound appointments were scheduled with as much precision as the administration of the pills and the shots. On this round of fertility treatments, and much to the doctors' and nurses' delight, the day of my final follicle measurements fell on a Sunday. Doctors and nurses love coming in on Sundays for ultrasounds.

Winnie greeted us, and Dr. New York the Man did the Sunday ultrasound, which didn't bother me as much this time because our follicles had grown last time, so I now assumed he was good luck. The room was a small, after-thought kind of room, but the setup was the same: table, stirrups, ultrasound wand (which is such a pleasant name, like it's magic and couldn't possibly cause any discomfort to my vagina), and big screen. The ultrasound was fast, and the picture that flashed on the screen dazzled our eyes.

"Seventeen centimeters!" Dr. New York proclaimed.

"Seventeen!" I repeated. We'd never made one that big!

"You'll be ready for the Giant-Stick-in-Your-Butt Shot tomorrow morning. You can do that one at home, too—"

"*No!*" Maybe I shouted it a little too quickly, in a way that somehow implied that I didn't trust my husband with the longest needle in the world. "I mean, I would rather a nurse do that one."

Both Winnie and Dr. New York set their pens down and looked at me. Phillip lowered his head. I started explaining. "No, no, he did a great job with the other shots. I mean, there was that little mishap with the wrong needle and almost puncturing my spleen, but we're over that now and I totally trust him to—"

Winnie laughed. "It's fine. Just come in tomorrow morning, and we'll fit you in."

"Thanks," I said with a relieved sigh.

This was the Giant-Stick-in-Your-Butt Shot. It was the last step before we could actually try to get pregnant. It was the last thing we needed to do in a doctor's office. After that, it would just be us and nature. Nature had let me down before.

High fives on the way out. Believing eyes. They gave me confidence.

• • • • • • • • • • • • • • • • • • • •

My next appointment was scheduled for the following Monday morning, which happened to be Halloween. At the doctor's office, the spirit was festive. The receptionist greeted Phillip and me dressed like a 1970s rocker chick. These folks took their holidays seriously. I guess if you're looking at women's uteruses and ovaries all day, you long for a break from the norm.

The Wicked Witch of the West called my name and led us to the Ponte Vedra Beach room for my ultrasound. I carried the Giant-Stick-in-Your-Butt Shot in a cute little paper bag. While waiting on the table, I played guessing games in my head about who would be walking in to examine me. Harry Potter maybe? Chucky? A Kardashian?

Would you believe it was none of those? No modern media news story character on crack could have topped what I saw walk in the door. It was sperm. A grown woman dressed as a giant, five-foot-tall sperm. A human-sized sperm had come to help me get pregnant. Now, if that wasn't an ancient Chinese proverb, or at least a sign of good luck, I didn't know what was.

She sat down at the end of the table to perform the final ultrasound (just one last check before the trigger shot that would release all my eggs). I couldn't stay still because I was laughing out loud. She kept having to reposition her head from within the giant sperm's head to see out to properly perform an internal ultrasound. I hardly noticed how big my follicles were when they flashed on the screen because a sperm was the one describing them to me. When she finally gave me the thumbs-up (do sperm have thumbs?), I watched her long sperm tail drag behind her as she left the room. I'm pretty sure that's the most times I've ever typed the word *sperm*, so thanks to her for that.

Another one of my nurses, a demure Green M&M (Get it? I mean we're trying to make babies here!), came in all smiles. "You're ready to release your egg!"

There weren't a lot of responses that seemed appropriate in the moment, so I just stuck with the smile and a thumbs-up right next to my face.

"I might get woozy with the Giant-Stick-in-Your-Butt Shot," I warned her.

She smiled and assured me I would be fine. The Green M&M left for a few moments to let me get dressed and mentally prepared while she prepared the Giant-Stick-in-Your-Butt Shot. I reminded myself this was all mind over matter and that, as long as I made the decision not to pass out, I probably wouldn't.

The Green M&M came back and propped me up in a standing position against the table so that, if I fainted, my face would land squarely in the outline of my own butt on the exam table sanitary paper. Then she picked up the Giant-Stick-in-Your-Butt Shot from her little aluminum tray.

"No counting," I told her, closing my eyes. "Just do it."

She grabbed a hunk of my buttock beneath my skirt and shoved that thing in deep! It felt as if it went all the way down to my ankle, but within a few seconds, the pain was gone. I had survived the Giant-Stick-in-Your-Butt Shot, and I would finally have my chance to let nature take its course. (You know, after all the pills and injectable drugs and ultrasounds, *nature* could take its course.)

"Great job!" the Green M&M shrieked. "Wait twelve hours, and then you guys can give this a fair try!"

"Yeah!" I exclaimed, caught up in the enthusiasm of the moment. "We're going to give this a fair try!" We fist bumped.

And then I got nervous.

There had been *plenty* of instructions on how to take the pills, administer the injections, and follow the "doctor speak" about my progress so far in the cycle. But remember, I was the twenty-seven-year-old who had no idea there was more to making babies that all the things combining and—*boom!*—baby. Thus far, none of my normal equations had worked. And no one had told me whether there were certain things I needed to do to actually "try." I was too embarrassed to ask Elvira in billing if there was some trick to it all, so the second I got home, I went back to Google School. I know. I know what you're thinking. Bad choice, Erin. But was I was just supposed to wait and see? Leave it to chance? Nope, not this babyless control freak. That seemed way too risky.

First I googled "The best sexual positions for conceiving." Let me be the example for the class on this subject forever and ever: Never enter the word *sexual* into a search string. You will not be led to what you're looking for. I clicked away from that screen so fast, I felt like I was trying to keep the neighbors from knowing what those websites were called.

Next, I googled "How to get pregnant." Well, that was the hot ticket to the baby train right there. Hundreds of women had posted personal stories of how they got pregnant. Pillow under the back, legs straight up in the air, thinking positively, headstand, leaning to the side you ovulated on—it was all there. So I took every single one of them seriously and decided that, if this was all I had control over, then this was what we would have to do.

On this night, I ambushed Phillip as soon as he walked into the kitchen. And not in a sexy way: "We will be trying while I lie on my right side on a stack of seven pillows with my legs hung from the ceiling fan, and directly afterward, your job is to stand me on my head and hold me there for thirty minutes while leaning me to the left. Oh, and then think positively," I added. "Now, go." I pointed to the bedroom.

"Erin." He grabbed my hand. "Billions of women have become pregnant without doing any of those things. We will be fine."

"This is our *one chance*, Phil," I said, staring him down. There's that forever mentality again. I'm not pregnant, and this is the only chance I'll ever have to get pregnant. I was truly a master at ruining most any situation with my forever mentality. "We spent all this time and money getting an egg and now you have to fertilize it, and you've got *one chance*. We have to do everything in our power to get this right."

He let go of my arm. "Wow. Okay. Well, now I feel the pressure."

"Good. You *should* feel pressure. I mean, not the kind of pressure that might make it hard for you to perform," I said hurriedly, "but the kind of pressure that should impress upon you the importance of this day. This opportunity. This is the last thing we have to do. It's like the last level of Super Mario Brothers. Save the princess, Phil. Save the princess."

"I get it, babe. I know it's important. Everything is going to be fine. Let's just try to enjoy ourselves." He began walking toward the bedroom.

"Okay. And align your chi," I said, following him. "I read in a Yahoo chatroom that you have a better chance if you align your chi before you do it."

Phil didn't acknowledge me. Or the Yahoo chatroom advice.

Once we were there, in bed saving the princess, Phillip stared into my eyes and stroked my hair, and I stared back, whispering, "Do you think I'm leaning far enough to the right?" I mean *nothing* about this experience felt like sex. Of course, midtry I remembered that having an orgasm also proved to increase a woman's chances of getting pregnant, so I had to do *that*. It was the most mechanical orgasm ever. I didn't even have feelings, just physical reactions. How do you keep intimacy when all of a sudden sex is so purposeful? In short, you don't. At least not the first time you try.

CHAPTER 9

The Negative

We tried two more times over the course of the next two days. Then we waited. It was almost two weeks before we would get to take a pregnancy blood test at Dr. New York's office, so we decided to get one of those five-day early pregnancy tests and take it at home. Besides, once we took our blood test it would take five hours to get the results, and I couldn't imagine waiting that long. This way, even if the results were negative, we could be emotionally ready for the next day. Phillip wouldn't be home from work until six, so I had the entire afternoon to net raccoon-sized butterflies in my stomach and put them in a jar for wall art later.

I went to the drug store to pick up a test. I also needed a refill on the drug the doctor had put me on to help control my sugar. The thing was, I wouldn't be able to take it anymore if I was pregnant, so I went back and forth as to whether or not it was a good idea to refill the medicine. If I did refill it, it could jinx the test or scare away the positive result. If I didn't refill it, it meant I was so sure I was pregnant that I didn't even need the medicine anymore. If I did refill it, it might be like admitting I didn't think I was pregnant. If I didn't refill it, and I wasn't pregnant, then not only would I have the pain of not being pregnant, but I would also have to make another trip to the drugstore.

Finally, someone in the pharmacy department noticed I was just standing there staring at the yeast infection medications and asked me if I needed help. I refrained from asking what he thought I should do. I just grabbed a pregnancy test and headed back to refill the prescription.

I'm here. I might as well fill it, I thought. A lovely woman got my meds and looked me right in the eye as she rang me up. She smiled and said, "Congratulations, and good luck!"

Well, if "to refill or not to refill" wasn't enough, now I had "congratulations" *and* "good luck." *Which is it? Congratulations or good luck? I'm looking for signs here, lady. I need a clue. I'm seeing omens everywhere, and the best you can come up with is congrats and good luck? You couldn't just say one or the other? You had to say* both*? Because now you're making me rethink the brand of pregnancy test I bought, and if I bought the wrong one and the results are inaccurate, I'm going to sue you.*

I took a deep breath, thanked her, and left.

It took seven hundred and ninety-four hours for my husband to come home, but when he did, I immediately ran into the bathroom with the stick. I decided I would pee on the stick and turn it upside down. I didn't want to see anything that might confuse me. I flipped it and ran into the kitchen from the bathroom. "You read it," I said to Phil.

"Okay," he said as he started toward the bathroom.

"Not yet! You have to wait two minutes."

"Okay."

We stood in the kitchen together and stared at each other, me leaning on a stool and Phil leaning on the counter, waiting for two minutes. You've heard that's the longest two minutes ever? It's longer than that. It's a sixteen-hour flight to Australia taken immediately after waiting in line at the DMV on a Friday afternoon to renew your passport. I stared at the clock, Phil stared at his watch, and every fifteen seconds we glanced at each other to either look away or make a "Yuck, this sucks" face.

Finally, when my heart was beating so fast I thought I might pass out, the second hand on Phil's watch hit two minutes and he walked to the bathroom. I could hear him pick up the stick.

He sauntered into the kitchen slowly, test in his hand. I was breathing so fast I couldn't even feel my chest going up and down anymore. Finally.

"It says not pregnant," he said.

He almost smiled.

I'm not sure I responded.

I don't even think I looked at him after I saw him almost smile. I just sort of collapsed on top of a stool. I was simultaneously devastated that it was negative and incensed that my own husband almost smiled when we learned all that work was for nothing. Why would he smile? Why would anything about this be funny?

Men don't react the same way women do when a fertility treatment fails. Most of them desperately want to relate to what we're experiencing, but they know deep down they can't. So sometimes they get unreasonably angry. Sometimes they pretend as if nothing has happened at all. And, sometimes, they nearly smile because they're so uncomfortable facing their own inability to help or change the outcome.

"Are you sure?" I managed.

"Yeah."

I started waiting for the episode of *Friends* to play out when Phoebe tells Rachel her pregnancy test is negative, and then when Rachel cries because she's so sad, Phoebe tells her the truth (she *is* pregnant), and now Rachel knows how she truly feels about being pregnant. I looked at my husband for a minute, waiting for him to say, "I lied before! It's positive!" He never did. He just stared back at me with that weird smile.

The tears came and went about twenty times that night. There are no words to describe the pain I felt for losing something I never had, something I had worked so hard for. It just seemed like the path. This is the new life equation, remember? We start trying, I get diagnosed, we make a plan, I write a blog, and *boom!*

But no boom.

No nothing.

At one point, after enough crying, I got angry. I got angry that I hadn't done something right. I got angry that I couldn't have what I wanted. I got angry that my husband hadn't responded the way I thought he should.

"Why aren't you even sad?" I barked from the kitchen to the living room.

"I am sad," he said, slowly walking back to the kitchen because he knew I wasn't going to let up.

"You aren't showing it. You aren't even slowing down to think about it. You're watching TV. How is this not even affecting you? It seemed like you were smiling when you found out I wasn't pregnant. Do you even want me to get pregnant?"

"It is affecting me," he said. "I'm sad. Of course I am sad. I didn't smile. But we can try again."

"Not until we've mourned this time, Phil. We can't just move right along. We have to go through and feel all of it before we can just dive in again, blind and with all kinds of yucky feelings."

"Well, I'm sad," he repeated. "I am."

"You still look like you're smiling," I said.

"I'm not. Maybe I am. I don't know."

We didn't talk anymore that night. We didn't hug it out, and we didn't snuggle. We didn't do anything else together. I sat in the bedroom and watched TV until I fell asleep. I'm not sure what he did.

• • • • • • • • • • • • • • • • • • • •

The next morning, the entire doctor's office knew the second they saw me. My eyes were bloodshot, and instead of a perky little greeting, I just mumbled hello. Phillip didn't say anything. Pam's eyes met mine in the lobby when she called my name, and as I approached her I said, "We took a test."

"You did? Oh no! Did you take one of those five-day early tests?"

"Yes. I did."

"Maybe you drank too much water beforehand? Diluted the test?"

"No, I didn't."

"Well, there's still a chance that it was just plain wrong, honey." Pam sat me down for the blood test in the hallway between two exam rooms. I had to squeeze a squishy ball while she found a vein. And what was the squishy ball in the shape of you ask. A big squishy sperm, of course.

Phillip took the other two squishy balls—a bull and a ball respectively—and began a short circus show just for me so I wouldn't look at the needle. While the bull was trying to balance on the ball, I stared that sperm in the eyes (yeah, it had eyes) while I squeezed. For a moment, our gaze locked, and I said in my head to that sperm, "Listen. I am doing everything I can here—pills, shots, positions. The least you can do is swim. Do you need directions? A more clearly marked path? It's your only job, so I'd really appreciate it if you could figure out what you need to get the job done quickly and correctly. We're all counting on you."

Pam drew the blood before I could finish the conversation with the squeezie sperm, and she sent me on my way. I stopped and chatted with Winnie about how to proceed.

"Don't worry, sweetie," she said. "We can just start again."

"What do I do?"

"I'll give you another birth control ring, you'll get a period, and while we wait, we can order the next set of injectables."

"Should I be doing something else?" I insisted. "Something more?" I was despondent. Desperate. *What else could I do?*

"Let's not make any big decisions right now," she said, smiling. "We will plan out the next steps with the doctor after you start your period."

I was sick at the thought of doing all this over again. With perfectionism in one pocket and my own worst critic in the other, I was entirely dissatisfied with myself. We had gone full-blown fertility treatments on this last round. We'd done pills, ultrasounds, and injections. Now that I knew this round hadn't worked, there was no telling how many times we would have to do it all again.

The fear became so infinite, my sadness simply labeled having a child as impossible.

CHAPTER 10

Things I Started to Hate

I saw my parents fight one time when I was growing up. My mom used to tell me they had a total of only three fights during their entire marriage. They instead did what my mom used to call "dancing." When she could feel my father getting irritated or ornery about something, she danced around it with humor or redirection, and my father did the same. One day when he got home from work (and after my mother and I both ran to the front door to hug him), he sat down at the bar with a small glass of scotch and began to talk about his day. "And then, this kid walks into my office as though he hasn't been gone for three weeks asking for his job back!"

"Mmm, hmm." My mother listened as she chopped a green bell pepper across from him.

"Are you going to cut it on the diagonal like that?" my father asked her.

"Yes, why?"

"Nothing. Anyway, I looked at him and I said you've got some nerve even walking in here!"

"Right ..."

"Why wouldn't you cut it the long way?" he interrupted himself again.

My mother, a twinkle in her eye, gathered up the already-sliced bell pepper next to the unsliced bell pepper onto her cutting board, slid the knife on top, and pushed it across the bar. "Here, then. You do it." My father laughed, pushed it back, took a sip of his scotch, and went on with his story.

No outburst. No dredging up the past. Just a dance.

My mom said that dance is the key to marriage.

Phillip and I didn't fight. We talked. We talked a lot. Sometimes we talked too much about things that didn't really matter. Sometimes we didn't talk enough about things that really did matter. Instead of dancing with each other, I think we danced around each other, past each other. Instead of telling him I wanted him to cry with me, I told him I needed him to remember the tomatoes if they were on the list. Instead of telling me he was scared, he stayed at work a little longer. I know that, as time wore on, I felt more and more alone. I think he wasn't really sure how to make me feel less alone.

There is no escaping the pain of infertility. There is no dancing through the pain when you want a child.

There was no question that we would try again … again. It wasn't a conversation we needed to have. The question was whether or not we would try intrauterine insemination (IUI) or in vitro fertilization (IVF). These were, respectively, the next steps up. They both required more intervention—more physical intervention—and more money, but also a better chance of getting pregnant. It's a brain-splitting decision while you're making it. At this point, though, we both agreed we wanted to use the injectables again. We didn't have to decide the rest until we met with Dr. New York again.

I kept my magic birth control ring in for a week and then, viola, I got my period. Winnie told me to call as soon as I got my period so we could set up another calendar and order the next round of drugs.

Sally the Shot Nurse called and suggested we try a different set of injectables that would be less expensive. The difference was that *all* of these new injectables would be arriving on different days, so I traded a little money for a little inconvenience. While they were less expensive, they weren't something you could set on the counter and forget about like butter; they had to be refrigerated, remember? So I had to be very careful to schedule the deliveries to arrive while someone was home. But the Far-Far-Away Pharmacy had to order these new injectables from other pharmacies as well, so coordinating which pharmacies could send which drugs on which days was a little bit worse than trying to schedule twenty-something servers at the Olive Garden. (Mmm, Olive Garden.)

We were planning to spend Thanksgiving in LA, so I ordered the first box's arrival the day after Thanksgiving, and the second for several days after. I had it on my calendar, my husband's calendar, and even in my neighbor's calendar (in case our flight back from LA was late, and she had to come get the goodness off our doorstep). *No way* would these cute little vials of fertility goodness get lost or go without the loving embrace of my refrigerator for any longer than they had to.

When we were flying home, we got stuck in Dallas. I texted our neighbor to say we'd be late and to ensure "the duck had landed" and that "the duck was in their fridge." She didn't respond. My husband texted her husband. No answer. Finally, as we boarded, we both called them. Their phones were off. Had they stolen the fertility goodness to sell on the black market? And the moment I realized our neighbors were attempting to thwart our plans for a child, the flight attendant told us to put our phones away. *But our neighbors are stealing our babies!*

It was a long three hours while I sat and prayed that our neighbors hadn't killed "the duck" by leaving it out in the "sunshine." (Too many quotations? I'm just getting started.) *Oh, please, Lord, save the fertility goodness from our evil and untrustworthy neighbors who turned off our sprinklers for us after they got stuck in the "on" position while we were away, saving us hundreds of dollars from the Electric Authority.*

They are obviously terrible people.

When we landed, I immediately turned my phone on. Text message. Crisis averted. The duck had landed, and it was safe in their fridge. Trust restored. Do you love how I overreact? Everyone does.

The second box was due at four o'clock on a Monday afternoon, and I wasn't concerned. We'd already had our scare, so this would be smooth sailing. We were both home and had no plans. We waited patiently for the box to arrive. Four p.m. Nothing. Four-fifteen. Nothing. Four thirty. Nothing. No worries. The delivery service was probably just running a little behind with all the other *potentially life-changing deliveries!*

Four forty-five. Five. Five thirty. Nothing.

You can imagine this new round of panic. What if the drugs were lost indefinitely? Then we would have to reorder them using the money we would make from selling our kidneys, because how else would we pay for more of these drugs?

I called the pharmacy in charge of shipping. A tiger of a representative sprang into action and went after the to-remain-unnamed package delivery service. She told them I was diabetic and needed the "insulin" that was in the package delivered to me immediately. (Hehe!) It felt great to have someone on my side but *ridiculous* that all of my fertility goodness was experiencing stress on its way to me. Stress kills sperm! Don't you know that?

As it turned out, the package had been delivered to the wrong house on the other side of town because the driver was "new" and didn't know the "route" or how to read "addresses" on "homes." Well, you should have heard the pharmacy rep really rip her a new one. Luckily, the people who received our package noticed that they didn't need any fertility drugs that day and kindly called the unnamed delivery service. My pharmacy rep insisted the driver go back out there after hours, pick it up, and then redeliver it to me with plenty of time to spare for refrigeration. This seemed an impossible task, as the driver was already back in her comfy home for the night. And I thought it was amazing that she was able to find her home what with all those pesky numbers on the mailboxes and street signs getting in the way. The two argued until, finally, another delivery person agreed to work late, retrieve my package from the wrong house, and deliver it to me before the ice melted along with our dreams of pregnancy. All parties agreed and, in fact, the "package" was delivered "safely" to my "porch" by seven.

• • • • • • • • • • • • • • • • • • •

I went to see a chiropractor before this next round began. My Google Doctorate provided me information regarding chiropractics and fertility. A Yoda of sorts, this chiropractor was giving me great hippy dippy advice for getting pregnant, which I loved. Aromatherapy. Sleeping positions. Herbs. With her long, muscular arms convincing my lower spine to move, she said, "Maybe you could try reading some nutritional websites. There might be alternatives to medication for getting pregnant you could try."

Face down on the table, I nodded. "If there might be a healthier alternative to eating bacon and ribeye for dinner every night, I'm in."

When the session was over, I went home and began googling. For those who've been playing along at home, you know this could have led to only confusion and panic.

These nutritional websites were all horrified at what I was eating. Without actually saying a word, they all basically guaranteed I'd be dead in a month if I kept up this animal product diet. This indicated to me that I needed to get pregnant within a month.

I read that dark legumes, sprouted wheat, blueberries, and kale were all I should be eating to cleanse my body of the animal tissue. This went against *everything* my endocrinologist had said (and, frankly, I still wondered where cheese fit in). I decided to keep eating meat and talk to the nurses at the endocrinologist's office about the internet's advice.

I went in for a precycle visit to make sure everything was fine before we started the whole process over again. This would be round three.

"So, Winnie," I said casually after my first ultrasound that ensured my blank slate, "I started reading some nutritional websi—"

I hadn't even finished the word before Winnie dropped her pen. Her eyes widened with betrayal. "Have you gone off your diet?"

"No, but I did read that—"

"I've have written letters to many websites on the internet that claim what we prescribe doesn't work," Winnie said gravely. "They do *not* understand that our goal here is to—"

"No no, Winnie," I interrupted. "It's fine. I'm not going to change anything about my diet." *I mean, I'm not going to change anything about my diet now that I've watched your eyes turn red and your hands start to shake at the mere mention of the words* nutritional websites.

"Okay, yes," Winnie said in a whoosh. "No, I know you wouldn't. You're not stupid, Erin. But some of my patients might have given into that crap."

Great. Now Winnie was mad at me. I would have to backpedal and backpedal fast. I quickly lied through my teeth, denouncing everything I'd read in favor of eating all animal products all day every day for the rest of my life to please her. These were the people I should be trusting anyway, right? They were the ones who had got hundreds of women pregnant before me! But I couldn't help but question whether my all-bacon diet was working. Ultimately, I decided to write out the pros and cons:

Pros with the endocrinologist: This diet had worked many times, and many women got pregnant this way. I'd seen the pictures of babies on the walls as proof.

Cons with the endocrinologist: Eating an all-meat diet could cause me to die of a heart attack.

Pros with the nutritional websites: I could enjoy a larger variety of food. And life would be more fun 'cause ... no heart attack!

Cons with the nutritional websites: There's no real evidence that his method will get me pregnant because there are no pictures of babies on walls.

Ultimately, my biological instincts to reproduce were much stronger than my fear of mortality, so I decided to stick with the endocrinologist's diet. And if I die before I finish this book, you'll know to trust the nutritional websites if *you* are trying to get pregnant.

• • • • • • • • • • • • • • • • • • •

I hated my diet. I felt far away from my husband. I couldn't get pregnant. And I was angry a lot of the time.

Like, how sick was I of hearing about women who "accidentally" got pregnant? It wasn't their fault, and they certainly shouldn't keep it a secret, but it sure did twist the knife when they remarked how terrified they were when they *found out* they were with child. It was unbelievably annoying when they told me they weren't even trying or didn't feel ready. *Yeah, you've been inconvenienced by a* person *you* made. *That's about the best freakin' inconvenience I can think of.* (Ironically, both my husband and I had been "surprises" for our parents. Did two accidents combining make a couple infertile? Was it like two like poles of a magnet? Our egg and sperm looked at each other like, "Oh, no. We will have *no more accidents.*")

And how about that TV show dedicated to people who didn't know they were even pregnant before they gave birth? Really? You didn't know? How adorable. You gained twenty pounds, puked, stopped your period *entirely*, became irretrievably moody, and started going into labor before you figured out that you were harboring life. You know what? Give me your baby. Just give it to me. If you didn't even know, what's the difference? You won't miss it, and then I'll get to have the baby I've always wanted. There should be a call-in number at the end of that show where infertile women can vote for which babies most deserve new mothers and why. Because, if you don't give those babies to someone else, in twenty years they'll all be on *Nightline* talking about how they felt as if their mothers never even knew they were there.

Because they didn't.

But this ... this was my favorite. Everyone and her sister *was* pregnant. At least one person from every part of my life was sporting a baby bump, all in varying sizes. And they were all afraid to *tell* me. Sure, they eventually told me, but they tiptoed because they didn't want to "hurt my feelings." Well, that pissed me off even more. It would hurt my feelings if they were secretly shooting my husband up with anabolic steroids or stealing my fertility goodness from the fridge. It didn't hurt my feelings that people I loved were pregnant. I thought it was tap-dancing, booty-shaking, kiss-'em-on-the-face fantastic that people I loved were pregnant.

Now, let's *not* talk about how expensive their labor and delivery bills were going to be. Their babies were free.

When you're going through infertility treatments, it's worth letting the people close to you know what you can and can't handle. I wish I had. No matter how much our people love us, they're not mind readers. Some women want to know when their friends are pregnant, and others feel that they're getting repeatedly throat punched when they find out. Decide where you fit on the spectrum. And try not to get mad at anybody for messing up by telling you more or less than you want to know.

I bitched and bitched and bitched so much on my blog and to my friends that I started realizing that the art of bitching is not a personality flaw; it might be a survival mechanism. I'd spent years attempting not to bitch, attempting to "dance." I snuck around problems and avoided hard conversations because I never wanted anyone to be upset. But this ... bitching. Bitching felt really good.

• • • • • • • • • • • • • • • • • • • •

I knew what The Inejectables felt like. The Giant-Stick-in-Your-Butt Shot and I had already faced off. And I'd already felt the emptying effects of a negative result. The worst thing that could happen was the same thing that had already happened. But maybe something new was what would hurl us over the finish line.

We discussed both IUI and IVF with Dr. New York at our ultrasound after I took the first Egg-Growin' Goodness pill. The IVF procedure would require Dr. New York to surgically remove an egg from my ovary, inject it with my husband's sperm in a petri dish, and then (if the egg responded to the fertilization) surgically implant it into my uterus. But neither Phillip nor I felt ready for that. It seemed like the last resort before surrogacy or adoption. So he suggested we try IUI for this cycle. Remember that stands for intrauterine insemination. Basically, he would put Phillip's swimmers into a long, plastic syringe that one of the nurses would slide into my cervix and release right next to the egg. Instead of the swimmers following road maps and honoring stop signs, it's sort of like they'd ride on a bus that would shove them out the door at the right stop and roar away with the driver shouting, "North!" It's also known as "artificial insemination."

Some may have thought it was premature to move up a level in the game of fertility. But I had just learned about bitching. I was ready to continue growing as a person.

Chapter 11

Cancel the Appointment

Good news: big follicles at the first ultrasound on the third round! And just with fertility pills!

I wrote a cheer for them:

Who's got fertility?
We do, we do!
Who do?
We do!
Goooooooooo fertility pills! (Kick one leg, one hand on
hip, while other reaches to the sky.)

I always wanted to be a cheerleader. Anyone who really knows me knows that.

After a strong week at Pilates, which I'd rejoined with vigor in this third cycle, my abs were pretty tight. I took a deep breath, closed my eyes, and Phillip poked me with the regular old needle. It burned, and I squeaked. When he pulled back I asked, "Done?"

"Nope." He held up the needle. It had *bent* trying to go into my skin. That's right. *Bent.* If you didn't believe in Pilates before, you believe in it now. Knowing what he now knew about the screw-cap needles, he simply attached a new needle and replunged.

For three nights, Phillip shot my belly, tracking the sites in the shape of a smile beneath my bellybutton. By the end, it looked as if a leprechaun had attacked me repeatedly with a Lilliputian's sword. What a leprechaun was doing with a Lilliputian's sword, I'll never know. I just hope the land of Lilliput isn't being threatened by leprechauns again. It just seems they should be on the same side.

After those three nights, my ultrasound gave us another reason to cheer: once again, the follicles had grown bigger. One was eighteen (translation: ready to go!), and one was fourteen (translation: ready to go in just a minute!). Turns out that my left ovary made more magic than my right one. This was sad because I'm right handed. I was sure my right ovary was sitting in there thinking, "All the *other* right-sided limbs and organs get to do stuff."

With all this action, Pam decided it was time for the Giant-Stick-in-Your-Butt Shot again. Things were different this time around because we were doing the IUI (artificial insemination). We had to time the Giant-Stick-in-Your-Butt Shot a perfect twelve hours before the IUI procedure. If we did it too early, we'd be getting inseminated at three o'clock in the morning, and I was pretty sure the nurse doing it at that time wouldn't be as accurate as the nurse doing it at ten in the morning. And if there's one thing you want when you're getting inseminated, it's an accurate nurse.

I sat at the edge of the exam table, ready for my next steps. Before Pam gave me the Giant-Stick-in-Your-Butt Shot schedule, she pulled out the Big Needle to show Phillip how to do the injection.

"Um, Pam," I interrupted. "Remember? I come *here* to get the Giant-Stick-in-Your-Butt Shot. He doesn't do it."

Pam laughed. "Not at ten o'clock at night you don't."

"Wait, are you saying the only time I can take this shot is at ten o'clock tomorrow night?"

"Well, yeah, if you want to attend your own IUI at ten the next morning."

"Who's going to be here at ten o'clock tomorrow night, Pam? Who?"

My face, mostly comprised of my saucer-sized brown eyes at this moment, stared Pam down like a mean girl in high school. Pam looked at me, more confused than frightened, and made the same face.

My husband took my hand and hushed me. "It's fine. I can do it."

"You cannot do the big shot. You *bent* the last *little* needle you tried to stick in me."

In hindsight, I'm not actually sure why I was so against Phillip giving me that shot. Yes, it was a bigger needle, and also an incredibly important step in the process (it released my eggs so they could be fertilized). But my common sense was slightly skewed by this point; my baby tunnel vision left no room for error.

I rushed home from our ultrasound with Pam and called my sister-in-law Sharon. She used to give flu shots back in the day when she worked in a doctor's office. At least she had some kind of medical background. Mind you, she also had a four-month-old baby at this point, but did that enter my mind when I asked if I could crash her house at ten at night and get her to shoot me in the butt? Well, yes. It entered my mind about an hour later when I was sitting on my bed sobbing hysterically over what a selfish, infertile girl I was. My sister-in-law immediately told me she would do the shot for me, of course. But I knew that, if I woke that baby up, it could screw up her entire night's sleep. And ruining that night's sleep meant possibly throwing off the rest of her *week's* sleep! That would have been on *me*. My emotional state was about as stable as a pony on a pogo stick, so I didn't think I could handle being responsible for a family's entire week's sleep.

Then I suddenly remembered the day Pam delivered my diagnosis to me right after inviting me to join the German American Club up the street from our house. Pam lived within a mile of us! She was always telling us to stop by! I wondered if Pam would mind if we stopped by at night? Say, ten o'clock at night?

I called Pam at the office to see what she would think about shooting me in my butt at night at her house. She didn't call me back until four that afternoon. (As if she had other patients?) She started out by giggling that she was usually in bed by nine. This was obviously her way of politely telling me that she didn't *want* to do the shot. But she hadn't said no yet, so I kept pushing in a disgustingly sweet way until she finally invited me over.

I called my husband to tell him the good news: "We're making a baby, and I don't need you for *anything* because I called Pam!"

Note: If you ever have to tell your spouse this bit of news, make sure that you tell him in a completely opposite way from the way I told mine. They don't tend to take it well when they learn they aren't needed for the process of making a child.

"Why can't you trust me to do this shot?" Phillip asked, surprising me with his hurt tone. "I realize it's scary, but I can handle it. I can do the shot."

"I'm sure you can do the shot, sweetie, but you don't have to! Pam can!"

"But I *want* to. I want to have a part in all of this. What else can I do?!"

"Well, you can go with me? You can hold my hand when she sticks me?"

He sighed. No more words.

I had a very minor feeling of regret when we hung up. I didn't want him to feel left out of the process. I'd already played out so many scenarios, though, in which having Pam give me the shot was imperative. What if Phillip's needle missed by even a few centimeters? What if he dropped the vial? My fears weren't off the wall, at least to me. I knew he wanted a baby as much as I did. I knew he didn't want any mistakes or setbacks. Why couldn't he play by my rules considering I was the one being ultrasounded and poked day in and day out? My feeling of regret turned into anger. *This is my body. This is my body going through hormonal swings big enough to clear the top deck of a cruise ship. I decide who gives me the shots. Period.*

• • • • • • • • • • • • • • • • • • •

After getting the Giant-Stick-in-Your-Butt Shot at Pam's house, in her bathroom, next to her husband's toothpaste, I got a good night's sleep. My husband's call time at the doctor's office was nine in the morning. Mine was ten. He had to make and leave a sample in a little room I liked to call Sample World. The doctor would then take the sample and "spin it down." This is technical speak for "spin it around." Dr. New York would pick the best, strongest, most Iron Man sperm of the bunch and put them into the really long, flimsy plastic syringe. And that's when the magic would happen. Or, at least, the magic would be injected into my uterus.

I was really excited.

Seeing as how he was hardly involved in the process of making the baby, Phillip was not enthused about his one contribution of marching to Sample World alone and leaving the lonely little cup for only the nurses and docs to see. He wanted me to go to Sample World with him. As Sample World was right there in Dr. New York's office, it only made sense that I should join him. But I couldn't stand the thought. First of all, I would have to have to *ask* someone if I could go into Sample World with my husband.

I couldn't just sneak in. This felt like high school when you asked if you could go to the bathroom right after your boyfriend three rows over asked. The teacher *totally* knew you were going to go make out, but you did it anyway. Second, assuming I got the green light to enter Sample World, I would have to actually go *in* there with him? This grossed me out because, *How many guys had been in there doing that in Sample World?* Presumably, *all* of them! I guess that, for guys, it isn't as freaky, but it's all I could think about. And third … well, third, it's Sample World, damn it. That's third.

Phil looked at me seriously and earnestly. "Babe, I at least want you to be there when," he paused, "the sample is made."

I knew I had to suck it up. When Winnie waved me back to get a quick ultrasound before the fun began, I told Phillip to stay in the waiting area. I couldn't ask her about going into Sample World in front of him.

"So!" I said, with faux nonchalance and cheer. "How's this all going to go down?" I hopped up on the table and slipped my feet in the stirrups as quickly and easily as I might put on a bra or untie my shoe.

"Well," Winnie said, equally brightly as she started the ultrasound, "he'll go first, and if you want to go home, you can. Otherwise, you can just wait until we're ready for you."

"Great." I nodded. "Great. So, I'll probably just surf the internet in the lobby. I don't want to drive all the way back home and risk getting stuck in traffic. Can I go with him to leave the sample? I might run downstairs and get a snack before you call me in if that's okay."

(Slick?)

I secretly hoped Winnie would say that it was forbidden for girls to enter Sample World. (When did samples go from being the best thing about Costco to the worst thing about baby making?) But, alas, Winnie almost whispered, "Sure. You can go with him."

Mortified, I found Phillip in the waiting area and told him that I could go to Sample World with him. He was very pleased, as noted by his modest grin and head nod.

Someone new called his name, and we marched back to the boy side of the fertility office. A large, Santa-like man dressed in scrubs escorted us to the very end of the hall where Sample World loomed. We all walked inside, and he closed the door. I looked around briefly and saw a wine-colored leather chair, a TV, a urinal, a toilet, a sink, and a clipboard. Very romantic.

Santa, who was very matter of fact, asked, "I assume that you're staying in here?"

I realized he was referring to me, turned bright red, and said "Yes" as professionally as if I was being interviewed for a high-paying job. I may have even adopted a British accent quite suddenly. I figured that would make this less awkward.

"Okay. Well, if you're staying here, there are some things I need to tell you."

Oh, God, please no. No things.

"First of all, you need to record the time the sample was taken. There's a clock on your clipboard."

Okay. Fine. I could do that.

"Second, you need to record it on your sheet if any of the sample is spilled and where it is spilled."

I was going to vomit *right that second* if I couldn't figure out how to disappear first.

"And third, since you've never done this together before, you need to talk beforehand about who is going to hold the cup."

I'm pretty sure my husband grabbed my arm to keep me from fleeing the scene when Santa opened the door to leave. "No problem," Phillip said.

It was … awkward. It was … weird. It was clinical. And strange. And very unsatisfying. And I had to take notes.

I won't go further into details except to say this: I realized partway during our time in Sample World that the excitement, the passion, the pure enjoyment that "leaving a sample" used to produce was all but gone. We weren't having regular sex for fun. We weren't being playful in Sample World. I didn't even feel as if we were attracted to each other anymore. I pushed past those thoughts and feelings to show up for Phillip.

In hindsight, I wish we had focused more on each other during this time as opposed to getting pregnant. Having a child was, of course, important, but it wasn't more important than fostering the relationship between the child's parents. But it's easy to get lost in it all when you're going through it.

If the before-the-sample portion of this day was mortifying, the after-the-sample portion was torture. Listen, on any other day, leaving that cup wouldn't make a difference. But knowing that this was the only link between "we don't have a baby" and "we do have a baby," it felt horrible just leaving it there on a little table. I wanted to tell someone to take very good care of it. I wanted to ask if they could pay close attention to the way they treated it and if I could be there when they spun it around so I could make sure they didn't mix it up with someone else's. I walked back to the lobby and thought about all the things I should have said to that little cup: "Listen, guys. You are strong. I know you might not have taken swimming lessons, but you are naturals. I know it. And I believe in you. If I may, though, I'd like to give you some guidance. First, swim up and to the right. My left, your right. That's where the egg is. Second, the egg is small, but it will look huge to you. There is a smaller one behind it. Either one is fine. Third, when you find the egg, do whatever it is you're supposed to do when you find the egg. I'm not really sure if you kiss it or hug it or offer a game of checkers. Just do the right thing. And we'll be cheering you on the entire time. I set you *free*! Now get out there and *swim*!"

While we waited in the lobby, another couple walked in. They signed in and sat down. Then the nurse called the man's name, and the couple walked back toward Santa. I chuckled to myself, knowing exactly what they were about to go do. I wanted to shout, "Don't forget to hold the cup and write down the time!" When they came back a few minutes later, it was strange to sit in the room with them. We all knew why we were there. We could all just talk about how silly this felt, but instead we sat there silently, trying not to make eye contact and exchanging low-toned conversations with our partners. Oh, well. Maybe the lobby of the fertility clinic isn't the first place people want to find friends.

After twenty minutes of awkwardness, Pam popped her head into the lobby. "Erin?"

I stood up and smiled. Phillip rose beside me, taking my hand.

"Ready, girl? This is it!"

"I'm ready!" I sang back.

We walked back to the girl side of the office where Pam led us to "New York City." She giggled and said, "If you get pregnant, your baby will be a New Yorker!" I thought this was very funny.

I lay down on the bed. Phillip read a business journal while he waited with me. Of all the different scenarios I had envisioned for the conception of our first child, this never even make the long list. Not that I had a whole *scene* pictured, but this was so casual, so … just another day at the office! I wanted heightened anticipation. Awareness. A feeling between Phillip and me that *this was it.*

Winnie popped in. She seemed to be laughing at a joke she had just heard. She was so thrilled to be the one who got to inseminate us. She talked and joked and hopped around the room, and I didn't really hear any of it. I felt sort of Zen. Super focused. Almost as if I was in the zone. The Baby Zone.

Winnie grabbed a long, floppy syringe in a package and held it up. "Sir," she said to Phillip, Winnie-seriously, "is this your name and social security number?"

"Yes, it is."

"Erin, is this the guy you want?" She showed me the package. There they were. The swimmers. I read Phillip's name, and since I've never been able to memorize his social security number—not even the last four numbers—I couldn't tell the difference between it and the formula written beneath it indicating the number of swimmers inside the syringe.

"That's him," I said. "What's that number?"

"Oh! That's his count! Twenty million!"

I looked at him, and he looked at me. "Twenty million, babe!" I exclaimed. "Wow, look at you!"

He smiled sheepishly.

"That's a great count!" Winnie chirped. "We are in *good* shape!"

I lay back, and she readied the tools. "Oh, Erin, you have such a beautiful cervix."

"Wow. Thank you." And before I could make a face at how silly that sounded, she was finished. It was just that quick.

"All right! Now relax for a while. You don't have anywhere to go, do you?"

"Nope. I'm hanging out," I said. I picked up a magazine, and Winnie cleaned up her supplies. She stopped short and said, "Whoa! What's this thing?"

"Oh. That is a fetish my friend Tamara gave me," I replied. Before grabbing the magazine, I'd retrieved it from a little pouch on my keychain. It was of southwest Native American origin, a miniature carving of a turquoise elephant.

"What's a fetish?"

"I'm not really sure." I shrugged. It was supposed to be imbued with a spiritual force, but I never asked Tamara how. "It's some kind of carving that represents health, and if you face it toward the east, it encourages fertility. She gave it to me for good luck, and I figured it couldn't hurt."

Just then, Sally the Shot Nurse popped in to check on me.

"Sally!" Winnie exclaimed. "Erin's all hippy dippy! Look at her little thing to help her be healthy and pregnant!"

"Oh, wow!" Sally picked up the fetish and set it back down facing the proper direction. "I didn't know you liked this stuff! Hold on!" Sally ran out of the room and seconds later returned with a fertility god made out of wood. "Look! We had this in the other room! We'll put this one in here too."

Then Winnie jumped. "Oh wait! That one ... the um—"

Sally interrupted. "Oh, right! With the thing! Hang on!" They both ran out of the room. I looked over at the fertility god and then the elephant fetish. One of them winked, for sure. The girls ran back in.

"This one is the 'Poof! You're Pregnant Fairy.' I'm going to poof you with it and then set it by your head."

"And this one is another one of those fertility gods. I don't know from which tribe or whatever, but it looks like a penis, so I'm sure it couldn't hurt."

"And this one ..."

They went on to describe and explain each little fertility god, fairy, and statue. They carefully placed each one in different places around the room and around my head. Phillip had to leave shortly thereafter for a meeting, and the girls had other patients, so I was left with all my new little friends. I had a huge smile on my face. Not to say that this was better than the normal method of conception, but I sure was stress free.

•••••••••••••••••••••

A week after our insemination and the morning before our blood test, Phillip kept delicately reminding me to take a pregnancy test. "You know, if you want to take one before the blood test, now would be the best time."

I knew he was right, but the anxiety I felt rivaled what Monk feels when faced with a communal pencil. I was absolutely paralyzed with fear.

The pain I'd felt with the last negative result had been so great and had lasted so long, I didn't think I could do it again. Of course, this was silly because I would inevitably have to experience another test result. The truth was, though, that I was pretty sure I wasn't pregnant. Even with the last cycle, I felt all kinds of shifting and feelings and sparklies in my tummy. This time I felt *nothing*. No sparklies, no nausea, no exhaustion.

Nothing.

When it was time for Phillip to leave for work, he made one last ditch effort to get me to take a test. "We have one in there, and we can just do it and get it over with and then get on with the day. Maybe it's positive?"

"I can't. I just can't," I responded without looking at him. He left, gently, and I stood alone in the kitchen.

Around one thirty that afternoon, I had two more phone calls and an inbox full of "I need" and "Can you?" messages. I was plugging away at my to-do list like Erin Brockovich on crack. Saving the world, one email at a time. It felt good to be so needed and to have so many people relying on me. For the first time that day, I felt as if I was on a roll. I was in a good place. I had a conference call in twenty minutes, and something said, "Go take the test. Do it right now and get it over with." I don't know who said it, but I'm sure my husband would like to know. He would call that voice all the time and be like, "Can you *please* ask my wife to close the kitchen cabinets that are level with my head when she's finished putting away the dishes?"

I ran into the bathroom. This was a fancy-pants test. I had to pee in a cup, use a dropper to get four drops, then drop them into the round space on the test stick. I peed (carefully) into the cup and set it on the counter. Remember that scene in *The Fifth Element* when Bruce Willis has to light the last match in his possession to open up the Fire Element Stone, therefore activating Leeloo's Love Element and saving the world from the meteor? That's exactly how I dropped the pee onto the stick. So carefully, so slowly, my eyes closer to pee than they'd ever been. It called for four drops. I would give it *exactly* four drops in a perfect, two-second-delay-between-each-drop kinda way.

When I was finished, I walked into the bedroom, sat on the bed, and breathed deeply.

I looked at the clock. It had been a minute.

I think I was supposed to wait for two minutes. Or, shit, was it three? Now I couldn't remember. The box was in the bathroom, and I couldn't look at the box without looking at the test. *I guess I'd better wait for at least two minutes. Or just go look now. I'll just go look now. I'm going.* I ran into the bathroom and looked down at the test.

There was nothing in the square indicator box.

Maybe nothing means pregnant, I thought.

I grabbed the box. I looked at the two examples on the front.

Empty indicator box clearly means not pregnant.

And two minutes was the wait time. It had definitely been two minutes by now.

Not pregnant.

I walked into the kitchen and cried. It didn't feel good, so I tried the living room. No better. I cried in every room until I was back in the bathroom, just in case it was tricking me and now read positive. Nothing. Empty indicator box. Not pregnant. And now I had a conference call in fifteen minutes. Awesome.

I barely got through my conference call without crying. I called Phillip afterward and told him I took a test without him and I was sorry that I did that, but the voice told me to, and it was negative like we thought (all in one breath). He was sorry and sad.

"Well, we'll try again next month," he said.

Since his parents were already with him, he went ahead and told them. That meant the entire family would know by the end of the hour, so I decided that meant I should tell my family too. I sent a quick email to those I knew would be waiting to hear from me. Quick like removing a Band-Aid. My message was short and to the point. I worked the rest of the day and ate a lot of chips. And bread. And chocolate. And drank wine. And I might have soaked a green olive in some vodka before eating it.

"You know, this could be a much longer process than we anticipated, and we should be ready for that," Phillip said to me, watching me soak another olive.

"I know," I answered quietly.

"Maybe we could consider adoption if we want a child sooner than later. Or maybe we could even talk about in-vitro fertilization, since I know that's pretty successful."

"I guess I'd rather adopt. I already feel like a pin cushion."

"Well, we could do that. We could decide how to do that. Together."

We agreed that eventually, somehow, we would have a child. It was hard thinking about adopting a baby and never being able to have our own baby, but the "baby" part was so much more important than the "own" part. Besides, every baby show on TV told stories of women who tried for three, four, even ten years before conceiving.

It was the strangest feeling, this conversation. It was a business negotiation. It was a heart-breaking corporate conversation. Was I willing to compromise my DNA to love another human as mine? Could I accept someone else's child? My emotions drained out of me while I mulled these questions over. It hurt too much to have emotions anymore. Facts. Facts were all I clung to.

The next morning, I begrudgingly went to my blood test at the doctor's office. I tried to sing along to the radio while envisioning having to make this very drive hundreds more times than I wanted.

When they called my name, I walked toward to the "blood station," and the nurse asked, "Sooo … what do we think?"

"I cheated," I said flatly. "I took a test. It was negative."

"Well, those tests are wrong all the time. You never know!"

"Yeah, well, it looks like my period is about to start, and last month we took a test on the same day and it was right."

She sort of frowned. I hate it when nurses frown.

Phillip wasn't there with me this time to put on a puppet show with the squeezie sperm and bull, so the needle really hurt. The nurse told me to go talk to "Scheduling" and come in for a consultation appointment. She said sometimes it feels good to go back to the drawing board and come up with a new plan. I couldn't imagine how many plans there could be. I mean, sperm, egg. How many combinations were there?

I told the gal at the front desk I wanted a consultation appointment with Dr. New York. She said that sounded like a great idea and offered me an appointment in two days.

I went home and ate more things I shouldn't and sat at my desk avoiding everything I needed to do. Feeling sorry for myself was the only thing that felt good. I forgot that I was getting a phone call in the afternoon to confirm the test results, so when the phone rang and I saw the fertility clinic's name on the caller ID, my heart got sad again. I picked up. "Yeah."

"Hey, sweetie, it's Sally. How are ya?" She said it in a sad, your-dreams-just-died-so-I-already-know-how-you-are kinda way.

"Oh, I'm okay, Sally. It's okay."

"Yeah. I know. Well, I went ahead and cancelled your consult appointment."

"Oh, okay. Wait, why?"

"Because you don't need it."

"Why?"

"Because you're pregnant."

PART 2

CHAPTER 12

You're Pregnant

"*Who* is? *Who* is pregnant?" I asked.

"You are!"

"I'm *not!*"

Sally laughed. "Yes, you are!"

"Whose file do you have in front of you?"

"Yours, Erin! Your file. You are pregnant."

"No, *I'm not!*"

Sally just kept giggling.

"Wait. Are you saying that *I'm* pregnant?" I asked. I was sitting at my desk in our home office. I leaned forward, setting my arm on the edge of my laptop, putting my face way too close to the screen, which made me squint.

"Yes, you are. You are quite pregnant."

"Okay," I repeated slowly, as if I were talking to someone to whom English was a fourth language. "So, I'm pregnant?"

This went on for quite a while. It was a wonder Sally didn't just finally shout, "*No, I lied. You're sterile. Shut up.*" Finally, I agreed that she had my chart in front of her, and that my chart said I was pregnant. Then the tears came. No, not tears of joy.

"Sally?" I stood up in front of my desk.

"Yes, dear?"

"I drank beer. And ate bread."

Sally laughed again. "It's okay, hun. Just don't drink anymore."

"Do you think I've hurt it?"

"No, it's fine. Don't worry about it."

I stood up and began pacing the house from home office to living room as she gave me the rundown of all the steps I should take: go off the pills that regulated my sugar, keep taking prenatals, refrain from taking any medicines that weren't on the list, and try to limit sugar as much as possible. Oh, and one more thing: pelvic rest.

Do you know what pelvic rest is? Let's just say you can't do anything fun that involves your pelvis. *Nothing.* No. Thing. There are no things you can do that involve fun and your pelvis. Are you getting my hint? Are you getting it? No salsa dancing. Now, I'd never been salsa dancing a day in my life. But it was just *agony* knowing that I couldn't start now.

Her last reminder to me was the date of my first ultrasound. "That will be your six-week mark. You'll come in, and we'll listen for a heartbeat and do a brief ultrasound. In the meantime, you'll need to take the pills that help you hold the pregnancy because you are automatically in the high-risk pregnancy category due to your infertility treatments."

I'd been given these pills during our first infertility cycle. That felt so long ago that I rushed to the medicine cabinet in our closet to find them while I was on the phone with Sally. She told me to take one each morning, and I agreed, rummaging through bottles and bags.

"Found them!" I exclaimed from the floor of the closet.

Once I hung up with Sally, I had to call Phillip. I had envisioned all these adorable ways I would tell him someday—serve *baby*back ribs for dinner with *baby* corn and *baby* carrots. Maybe do like my cousin did and put buns in the oven. Buy "It's a Girl" and "It's a Boy" balloons and string them in the hallway for when he got home from work. But I couldn't imagine keeping this secret to myself for the rest of the day. I couldn't tell anyone before I told him. And I was practically bursting at the seams. I had to tell *someone.* So I called him.

I decided to go back to pacing the house, except I added the kitchen to my path between the office and the living room. I waited almost nine months for him to answer. Finally ... "Hey, babe, what's up?" he said.

"Where are you?" I asked in a totally casual voice.

"I'm in Home Depot with my dad."

Oh, shit. He's with his dad. What do I do here?

"Oh, okay," I said lightly. "Well, Sally called."

"Oh." Phillip paused, and I could picture him in a cement-floored aisle, playing eenie, meenie, minie, moe with which tone of voice he should choose. He went with sensitive but strong. "You okay?"

"Yeah, I'm all right. She cancelled our consult appointment." I said it very matter-of-factly. I didn't smile or let my voice crack at all.

"Okay."

At this point, I wasn't sure if he was listening because he should have questioned that, but he didn't. Whatever. This was no time to start the "Are-you-even-listening-to-me?" nag session.

"Yeah, so she cancelled it because I'm pregnant." *Then* I smiled.

There was a pause. Then Phillip's voice came loud and strong and practically vibrating with joy. *"Are you kidding me?"*

"No." I smiled through the phone.

"Oh, my God. I'm going to cry in Home Depot!"

"Well, don't cry in Home Depot! Is your dad right there?"

"No, I ran to the next aisle when you called. He doesn't know where I am. Oh, my God. Are you sure?"

"Yep! Our home pregnancy test was wrong. Very wrong."

"Oh, wow. Oh, my gosh. I can't tell them right now. I'm not ready to tell the family."

"That's okay. You don't have to tell them."

"I know, but I have to finish installing a TV wall mount for them. I have to get it done today!" He was totally beside himself.

"Okay, go do it. Just come home when you're done."

"I can't install a tv wall mount right now! How am I going to do that?"

"I don't know! But you have to! Just go do it. It's okay. You can do it!"

So my poor husband spent the afternoon in his parents' kitchen installing a TV wall mount knowing all the while that his wife was pregnant with their first child. He couldn't focus. I kept getting text messages from him like, "I'm dying."

When he finally got home, we just stared at each other. Stared and said things like, "Wow" and "Holy crap." We wandered from one room of the house to another staring at each other and saying, "Holy crap."

I don't remember what we did that night. Probably just cooked dinner and watched TV the way we do on most nights. But I do remember that when we went to bed, he put his hand on my tummy and said, "G'night, Mama."

I giggled and closed my eyes.

CHAPTER 13

What-If Monsters

Our first instinct, naturally, was to tell *everyone*. We wanted to share the news with everyone we loved, everyone we knew—heck, even people we didn't like. But then the reality of all the different possible outcomes made themselves known by becoming angry little monsters in our heads. This specific breed of monster is called the What-If Monster. They remind you that, while this pregnancy is exciting, it is also very uncertain. They're kind of jerks.

As both a "fuck you" and a "yeah, you have some logic," to the What-If Monsters, we decided to tell our very closest friends and family. We kept a list of those we told in case we had to tell them that we'd lost the pregnancy. It was our biggest fear, but the What-If-We-Lose-the-Baby Monster made us face it.

A note: When you finally begin telling people you're pregnant with your first child, you assume they're going to jump up and down, throw hats and parties and streamers, be paint-your-face-on-a-billboard excited. And they are usually happy for you. But the way they choose to demonstrate that thrill lies on what I call The Reaction Continuum. Some people do scream and jump up and down. Some people cry the ugly cry. Some people remark, "Wow! That's excellent! After all that work!" And still other people look at you blankly and say something like, "Oh. Wow. Great." You can never predict what people's reactions will be, and it can leave you feeling a little, "Eff you for not being as excited as I am about my baby!"

We decided to call my mother and tell her over the phone because telling her in any way that involved the *least* amount of surprise would send her over the edge.

I called her the day after we learned the home pregnancy test was very wrong and laid it on her. "I'm pregnant." There was a disturbingly long pause. It was so long that I almost repeated myself, or whacked my phone and asked, "Is this thing on?" Finally, I heard a sniffle. That was my cue to pull the phone away from my ear. The woman cried one of those hit-the-floor, slam-your-head-into-a-wall, pound-on-your-knees-with-your-fists cries. It sounded like someone was eating her. But I knew it meant she was over-the-moon happy, so I let her cry it out. We didn't really talk about any of the details that day. I'm pretty sure I just told her I would let her go, and she wailed something into the phone before hanging up. Grandma was thrilled!

Then we told my sister-in-law Sharon. She responded in the way that she responded to most every piece of news we'd shared with her up until this point: "Oh you are? That's fantastic! I'm so happy for you." Simple. Honest. Not over the top.

We decided to tell Phillip's family in a fun and exciting way. So when his parents made reservations for the entire family to have dinner at the Melting Pot shortly after Christmas, about four days after we found out we were pregnant, we decided to make our move. We called the restaurant and asked that, after giving the family a rundown of the specials of the day, they also include the fact that we were expecting our first baby. Cute, right?

We walked in that night and double-checked with the hostess that everyone on the staff was in on the secret. She nodded knowingly, and we joined our family members in the bar while waiting for our table for fifteen to be ready. Once we were all led to our nearly private room and seated around a long, rectangular table, my heart started beating. This was the moment when everyone would raise a glass in the air and call for a round of "Hip-hip-hooray!" We would throw our heads back with laughter and, despite the fact that my belly looked just the same, everyone would still ask to feel it. We would clink our glasses and discuss which hospital we should use and possible names for a boy or a girl. I was so excited I couldn't stand it.

Then the waitress gave us the specials. " … and the special drink tonight is a dark chocolate mojito with strawberries in it. And Phillip and Erin are expecting."

She didn't even give the family a running start. I'm not even sure all of them heard her say it. And she said it with the least amount of gusto anyone has ever delivered that news with before, almost as if she didn't really understand what it meant—"expecting." Like maybe she just thought we were expecting … a surprise! Or a flash flood. Or a replacement credit card in the mail and we just wanted *everyone to know!*

The members of the family who *did* hear her turned and looked at us with looks of confusion, almost frustration. "Wait, what?" It took a full thirty seconds for the news to get around the table that, yes, I was pregnant, and, yes, we are surprising you with that news at dinner. By the time people figured out it was true, they were all on to ordering appetizers and—well—drinks.

So. It was a real memorable moment for us.

After we told all the people we wanted to tell, we had two weeks until our first ultrasound. Two weeks to wait at home and see if this pregnancy had actually "took." There is absolutely *no way* to convince a pregnancy to stay put. You'd better believe, if I had been singing to eggs before, I was singing to this little baby. "Come on, little baby, grow a heart! Make me fart! Come on, little baby, and hang on tight! With all your might!"

I had been four weeks pregnant the day I found out. (For you girls and guys who don't know, you count pregnancy weeks from the first day of the last period. My last period had started four weeks prior; hence, four weeks pregnant.) I had no symptoms aside from being a little more tired than usual. No neat pregnancy cravings. Nothing funny or surprising. And, of course, everyone said, "Great! You might be one of the lucky ones!" But I was thinking, *I would give anything to vomit all day every day, just to know I'm really pregnant.*

Phillip suggested taking a pregnancy test now that we knew we were pregnant just to prove it. I almost threw up with anxiety at the thought. The What-If Monster break-danced on my upper intestines. This vomit reaction, for a moment, quelled my fear that I wasn't pregnant. Until the nausea went away when Phillip said, "It's okay. We don't have to take a test."

I didn't.

Do you know the signs of a miscarriage? Odds are, if you've ever been pregnant, you know the signs. It's a huge What-If Monster that no one can prepare you for. The fear of never getting pregnant is dwarfed by the fear of losing a pregnancy once you actually achieve it. My What-If Monsters did take pleasure in enrolling me in Google Obstetrics class about six days after we found out we were expecting.

"How common is miscarriage?" I asked my benevolent instructor. "Miscarriage and PCOS," I amended, in case Google misunderstood the specificity of my question. "What are the signs of a miscarriage?"

If I've said it before, I'll say it again. Googling is a bad choice. *Bad* choice. I learned that my risk of miscarriage was almost forty-five percent because of PCOS. I learned that normal women have about a fifteen to twenty percent chance of miscarriage, and it almost always happens in the first trimester. I learned most miscarriages are due to chromosomal abnormalities, something moms have no control over. But women with PCOS have a higher incidence of chromosomal abnormalities because we just don't make good eggs.

Overwhelmed?

Yeah. I became terrified of having a miscarriage. I'm sure you're terrified of having one now, too, after reading that, even if you're a guy or not pregnant.

So I called Sally the Shot Nurse. I told her I'd just read on Google that I was going to have a miscarriage within the next two weeks and that I would likely never carry a baby to term without massive medical intervention. She gasped and immediately commanded, "Erin! No more Google! *Ever!*"

I agreed. Except ...

Unfortunately, I went to Barnes and Noble a few days later. I found a book about PCOS. The What-If Monster came snarling back into my life. Phillip encouraged me to close the book and read a funny high-risk pregnancy book. (Spoiler alert: there were no funny high-risk pregnancy books.) I said, "Okay," but I really meant, "Okay, I'll find a happy book as soon as I'm finished *completely freaking myself out with the scary book*." I proceeded to sit on the pregnancy section floor of Barnes and Noble and cry all by myself. Well, not all by myself; the What-If Monster was there, too, until Phillip came over and sat on him.

It was on this trip to Barnes and Noble that I learned there are a *billion* pregnancy books to choose from. A *billion*. I had already read several and decided to purchase a few that were recommended. If I can make a suggestion, never ever read any of these pregnancy books if you're prone to What-If Monsters. Please. Don't do it. Put them down. There are entire sections of these books that are actually written *by* What-If Monsters. It should be considered cruelty to women who live with What-If Monsters. Every possible thing that can go wrong is listed *in detail*, followed by, "Oh, but don't worry. I'm sure that won't happen to you." I had listeria and toxoplasmosis more times than I can count because of these books.

There are, of course, some good books out there. Not overwhelming, but just enough information to answer some basic questions. (Why am I completely constipated all of a sudden? More on that later …). I took solace in *Belly Laughs* by Jenny McCarthy and *The Girlfriends' Guide to Pregnancy* by Vicki Iovine. Phillip started reading *The Official Lamaze Guide* by Judith Lothian, a book a friend gave to us. The day he read a few pages out loud about how pregnancy is not a sickness and you can give birth without any intervention at all, I informed him that he was welcome to continue reading that book while I was getting my epidural.

Like everything, my decision to have an epidural would change. About nine more times …

My What-If Monsters kicked in big time when a girlfriend told me about her scare with Down syndrome. She explained that, because of her high-risk pregnancy status, she was also at higher risk for genetic imperfections resulting in diagnoses of Down syndrome, Fragile X syndrome, and other scary outcomes. When her nurse told her she needed to come into the office to receive the results of her testing, she was positive it was bad news. Her doctor simply wanted to tell her in person that all was well (cruel, cruel trick), but her happy ending had my What-If Monsters doing an amazing conga line of panic in my head. I was at high risk for pretty much *everything* it seemed.

And then there were, of course, the What-If Monsters that I created entirely on my own based on no facts and very little understanding of scientific facts. The overwhelming fear of my child getting stuck in my pelvis during the birthing process and then having to remove my bones and muscles to get my baby out (because how else would you do it?) was one of the most ridiculous. I also feared that my ankles would swell and never go back to their normal size, that stretch marks would totally disfigure my torso, and I would sustain permanent spine injury from carrying my front baby load. I feared food poisoning and what it could do to my baby. I feared having to get rid of my beloved dogs because perhaps my pregnant body might be allergic to them, and of course, I feared that the What-If Monsters might never go away.

Of all the ridiculous What-If Monsters, ridiculous dreams weren't even mentioned in any of my What-If Monster books or websites. But, oh, how they reared their ugly heads.

I've had some weird dreams in my life. And they usually pop up when I'm experiencing some great change or shift. But nothing—and I mean *nothing*—could prepare me for the vivid and insane dreams I started having after I got pregnant.

The first truly disturbing dream began with me sitting in the hotel that I owned and lived in. It was beautiful, and there were many carpeted staircases. When a certain woman checked into the hotel, I watched her from across the lobby. And I knew what I had to do. I had to stalk her throughout the entire hotel with the cunning use of a walkie-talkie (though no one was talking to me on the other end). I followed her all the way to her room and waited until she got in the shower. When I heard the water stop running, I immediately burst into the bathroom and cut off her head. I threw her body out the window and tossed her head in the bathtub to "clean it." Once I wiped up all the blood, I shoved her head in the ceiling fan and went back down to the lobby. You know, typical hotel owner day. (To clarify, I step over ants whenever possible so as not to squish them. Chopping heads off was way out there in left field.)

I dreamt that I laid concrete with Tony Romo while I was wearing a very pretty dress, saved Phillip from an earthquake in Paris by rocking him to sleep, and searched the city for empty buildings where Phillip and I could build a new room for the baby. It was maddening to wake up every morning and have to convince myself that I'd probably never met Tony Romo and that the lady from the hotel was more than likely feeling just fine. The only What-If Monster I really came away with was hoping Phillip would be able to get rid of his tail before the baby was born.

CHAPTER 14

Am I Losing It?

At about six weeks, I started feeling a lot more tired, and my normal love of food and cooking slowed down. I didn't feel nauseous, but I did feel angry with food and some of the smells it made. If Phillip cooked broccoli, I cursed him for hours. I could smell peanuts in other houses. However, if pineapple or peaches were within a five-mile radius, I could track them like a bloodhound and eat every last bite. Fruit tasted *so* good. Better than it had ever tasted before. I don't know what it was doing hiding among the produce because I thought it should be stored *in* the grocery store shopping carts.

I also started experiencing mood swings. I didn't often get angry, but I did experience most emotions fully. (That's a nice way to say it, huh?) Like the day Phillip and I decided we would begin repainting some of the walls in our house. The main color of the house had been a sun-shiny 1997 yellow when we bought it. I'd seen a muted, matte cappuccino colored wall in a friend's house and wanted our entire house to be that color. We went to Home Depot, chose something similar to cappuccino, and got me a handy-dandy little face mask so I couldn't hurt my baby with paint fumes. Phillip did most of the painting while I did most of the taping. Once the entire front hallway was complete, we took a step back.

"I like it," Phillip said.

"Me too!" I said, and we went on about cleaning up supplies.

About an hour later, I walked into the kitchen to get a snack, and Phillip asked me if I wanted some pineapple. I responded, "I really love the paint color."

"Me too, babe."

I went on, "No, I mean I really love it. Like, I'm just so happy about it."

"Good!"

Not finished. "It is just so pretty and exactly what we wanted it to be, and we are so lucky."

"Right. It's great. Do you want—"

I interrupted. "I just, I want you to know how happy …" The tears started flowing. "… how happy I am that we chose this color."

"Okay. Wait. Are you … are you crying about the paint color?"

"Yeah. Yeah, I think I am. I just love it so much."

Phillip stared at me for a few minutes while I cried about loving the paint to make sure I wasn't playing a trick on him or waiting for the staff members of Candid Camera to pop out of the living room. Finally, he gave me a hug, and in a sort of "What the hell is going on?" tone, he said, "Okay. Well, really good. So glad you like it. I like it, too."

I wiped my tears away, puffed out a few last sniffles, and proceeded to eat an entire pineapple.

· · · · · · · · · · · · · · · · · · · ·

Phillip continued occasionally asking me to take a pregnancy test at home. I thought about it a lot until I realized that if I didn't take a pregnancy test, I'd never have a picture of the positive test result. You know, the picture everyone has now, and they post it on Facebook and Twitter and email it to everyone they know, including ex-boyfriends? I wanted one of those pictures. I wanted that memory. So I decided we should take a test.

I woke up with a feeling of enormous fear in my chest. "What-If" I took this test and found out I'd lost the pregnancy? I couldn't handle that. I absolutely couldn't. I just wanted to see the two lines. I wanted it so badly. I forced myself up and out of bed, peed on the stick, and walked back to bed. Phillip was already up and getting ready for work. His routine was always the same. He made coffee and then he showered. Then he looked at himself in the mirror (occasionally shaving but usually just pretending like there was much more than that to do). Then he got dressed and spent the rest of the morning in the kitchen making an elaborate breakfast. It's his favorite meal, so he often spent fifteen to twenty minutes making the perfect bowl of oatmeal with crushed nuts and fruit, or perhaps an egg scramble using avocado, tomatoes, fresh spinach, and various cheeses. On this morning, once he was getting dressed, I told him to go in and read the test. I pretended to go back to sleep.

He didn't realize how scared I was. He didn't know my heart was beating out of my chest and I couldn't control my breathing. He couldn't have known, because he walked by the test on his way to grab a towel from the rack in the bathroom and said, "Oh look, it's done. You're pregnant."

In a relief-induced haze, full of endorphins, I walked from the bed to the bathroom and looked at it. It was true. The little lines on the pregnancy test, albeit really light, were there. The doctor said I was pregnant, and now this stick said I was pregnant. And, in journalism, for a story to be published as fact, you need two sources.

One.

Two.

• • • • • • • • • • • • • • • • • • •

At six weeks, I got to have my first ultrasound. Because I had got pregnant by way of fertility treatments, I was automatically labeled a "high-risk pregnancy." While nothing risky had yet happened, I would need to have weekly ultrasounds to track progress. On the morning of the first ultrasound, I woke up and tried journaling and reading good pregnancy books, but in the end, I couldn't kick the panic. Seeing as I'd had very few symptoms and only super-light lines had appeared on the pregnancy test, I just didn't see how there could really be a baby in there.

But then, the worst thing that could have happened did.

I took my mandatory wake-up-and-immediately-pee pee and found that I was bleeding. There was not enough blood to stain my underwear, but enough to show on the toilet paper. Blood. Blood means miscarriage. I sat on the toilet in shock, my heart beginning to beat too fast. I stood up, pulled up my underwear, and braced myself on the bathroom counter. Before I could even look myself in the eye in the mirror, my knees hit the floor. And I cried. I silently sobbed on the bathmat. "No, no, no," I repeated quietly. I took huge, long, sweeping inhales and pushed them on in short bursts, tears falling out of my eyes and hitting the bath mat.

I watched them. I listened to them hit the mat, almost outside of myself. *How can this be happening?*

Phillip had already left for work, so I was all alone. As soon as I could get myself off the floor, my first instinct was to immediately start googling or flipping through pregnancy books, but I was entirely too terrified. I walked from the bedroom to the bathroom, empty, out of control. It was the most awful feeling I'd ever felt. Here I was, six weeks pregnant after nine months of trying, and I might be losing the baby. It was almost too much to breathe through, but I knew if I didn't get myself dressed and to the doctor, I couldn't know for sure. And not knowing was much worse.

I stood for a moment in the closet, and I prayed. I prayed to my dad to please, please help this baby live inside of me. I prayed to him to be with me, to stay with me, to be my strength as I got to the doctor's office. I wrapped my hands around the edge of a shelf in my closet and tensed my arms, whispering, "Pleeease, Daddy. Please." And without warning, clear as though he were standing next to me in the closet, he said, "You're not losing the baby." On a huge inhale, I asked out loud while crying, "I'm not?" I did not receive another answer. Not another word. I didn't feel relieved or convinced, but hope suddenly and unexpectedly added itself to the equation.

On my way out the door, I felt as if my dad was pulling me back into our home office. I opened my computer to see if I had any important emails, as I couldn't imagine any other reason to be in the office, and there it was. My first BabyProgress email update. I had signed up for updates the day I found out I was pregnant, entering the date of conception and my email address. Each week, I received an email telling me about the size of my baby, information about development, and information about pregnancy at that stage. And there, right in black and white at the end of the paragraph, I read: "At six weeks, bleeding may occur. This can oftentimes be normal."

I let out a huge whoosh of air and swallowed hard. It was enough to get me into the car and on the road. Thanks, Dad.

Phillip was going to meet me at the office at our appointment time. I called him on the way to tell him what was going on, but I was brief, blunt, and emotionless at that point. I just wanted to know what was happening. When we met in the lobby, we both walked as if on a mission, neither saying a word. We didn't need to say anything to each other. We both just wanted to know if this was the beginning of the beginning or the beginning of the end.

Winnie saw me in the hallway and immediately changed her course with a huge smile and the makings of a hug to congratulate me. Then she saw my face and her expression turned from joyful to inquisitive. "I'm bleeding," I answered her face.

"Okay, let's go," she said, skipping the pleasantries and the possibilities in favor of an exam room. "Wait here. I'll get him."

Dr. New York was normally very prompt, but that day it seemed that everyone was busy, and no one could take the time to reassure me that everything was okay before I went in. It took an agonizing twenty minutes for Dr. New York to walk in the door, and he didn't even have a chance to say hi before I launched into explaining the situation and asking if I was losing the pregnancy. Understanding my fear, he skipped casual conversation. "This is really normal, Erin," he said as he set up the ultrasound machine. "My wife had similar bleeding with all three of her pregnancies." He moved through his comforting words so that I didn't have to wait a second longer than I needed to. He quickly put on his gloves, positioned the ultrasound wand, and here's what we saw: A teeny, tiny, white, ghostly lima bean. When the ultrasound machine zoomed in, the lightest little light—lighter than the positive pregnancy test—flickered. It flickered with life.

"Holy. Crap." I said it out loud.

"See that flicker? That's a heart," Dr. New York calmly but proudly showed us.

Phillip stood next to me recording the entire experience on video, saying factual things like, "That looks like a valve in the heart" and "It appears strong."

I just kept saying "Oh. My gosh" and "Holy. Crap." Because in times of stress or satisfaction—and especially when I experience both together—I'm inappropriate at best.

Dr. New York explained that bleeding at six weeks is often similar to a period for women and that it's not always a bad thing. It often means the egg has implanted; in other words, it has stuck itself to the wall of the uterus to hold on for the ride. And that egg, now my baby, was measuring the length of the lima bean that rested inside of a sac (which was actually a little halo around the egg that provided nourishment until it grew an umbilical cord). Phillip went on stating facts, and I went on with inappropriate comments until the ultrasound was over.

"There you have it," Dr. New York beamed at us. "That's a baby."

CHAPTER 15

Meeting my Midwife

The nausea and exhaustion were now obvious. It was like having a light flu for weeks with absolutely no medication and no relief. Whoever said that pregnancy is beautiful was a dirty liar.

I ate weird things at weird times, like spaghetti for breakfast. I also suddenly hated the smell of our couches until, after smelling around for quite some time, I realized it was actually the smell of our walls I hated. *Hated.* I felt physical sadness about our walls.

Have I mentioned the constipation? If somebody's going to tell you, it might as well be me. Never in my life had I experienced anything like this. And with all the fruit I was eating, I couldn't for the life of me understand how this poop was staying in there for *days.* I read in one of my pregnancy books that constipation could be so bad that women might actually consider using the breathing and muscle control techniques that are used during labor. *Labor.* For poop.

I also couldn't eat anything without falling asleep immediately afterward. A starving maniac every few hours, I would shove my face full of non-related foods and then fall asleep wherever I had finished eating. Sitting up. Leaning against a wall. It was a good thing I was working from home.

Getting up to go to the ultrasounds was the only time I ever set my alarm anymore. And it was pretty worth it every time. Eight weeks in, Dr. New York said a lot of times babies start to move at that point.

At my eight-week appointment, from the stirrups position, I asked him, "Are those arms? And legs?"

"More like hands and feet," Dr. New York responded. "But yes. They look great!"

"Is he going to move?" I asked.

"I'm not sure," he responded in a tone that made it clear he was more intent on measurements and vital signs than whether or not the baby would put on a show for me.

"If it's not moving, is it asleep?" Phillip asked, peering at the screen.

"Could be, yeah. Could just be still for now," Dr. New York said.

"Maybe he's in a coma!" Winnie chuckled.

Yeah. Never a good idea to joke with a newly expectant mother that her as-yet-unborn child is in a coma in her uterus.

"So everything looks okay?" I asked, my voice now slightly tinged with panic.

"Everything looks awesome," Dr. New York said as he began printing out pictures from the ultrasound machine and washing his hands. "We're right where we need to be and we'll see you again two more times before you can transition to your regular gynecologist."

The only very small problem with this last statement was that I didn't have a regular gynecologist. I didn't want to go back to that blonde bimbo who had cheerily told me, three weeks before her own due date, that I'd be pregnant in no time. So before I left the office that day, I asked Winnie and Pam whom I should see.

"Go see my best friend! She's a midwife in an ob-gyn's office. Her name's Annie. You'll love her! You'll just love her!" Winnie said.

"You're going to get a C-section, right? Just get a C-section. It's way easier," Pam added, half joking and half serious.

"I ... I don't know if I'm getting a C-section ..." I started.

"Oh, stop!" Winnie said. "Don't listen to her. Just go see Annie. I'll give you her number. She's my best friend!" she repeated.

"Well, if she's *your* friend, I'm sure I'll like her," I said.

"But seriously, think about getting a C-section," Pam continued as I walked away with Annie's card.

• • • • • • • • • • • • • • • • • • •

I made an appointment to meet Annie and determine if I wanted her to deliver my baby. Having never interviewed anyone for this position before, I didn't really know the right questions to ask. Have you done this before? How many times? What's your favorite kind of birth? Have you ever dressed up like a sperm to do an ultrasound?

Phillip went with me to meet Annie, and we were both immediately put at ease. Annie was a middle-aged midwife, no husband and no kids, and a real straight shooter. I ended up telling her more than asking her anything at all. After telling her about my infertility treatment, I explained to her that I wanted my pregnancy to feel as natural as possible. She completely understood why, after all my treatments, I wanted the least intervention possible moving forward. She also assured me that, while she would give me as much freedom as possible during my pregnancy, she would never allow me to make a decision that might put me or my baby at risk. She promised to listen to my concerns, and she reminded me that I knew my body best.

Her ability to look at all of this simply and with a chuckle made me feel that I could look to her to find out if I should be panicking or not. I felt that I could trust her reactions better than I could trust my own. That's what I think most of us should be asking our doctors, especially the ones who help us bring our babies into the world: will you listen to me and will you guide me?

I asked Annie what she thought about home births, hospitals, and C-sections. "I think your baby will probably come into the world on its own time and in its own way. But my goal is to keep you both healthy and safe."

"Right. Me, too. Are C-sections better?"

"There are pros and cons to all of it. I don't do C-sections because I'm a midwife. Our ob-gyn here in the office would do that. If you choose this practice, you'll work with both of us. And however your birth ends up, that will determine which of us helps you deliver."

"So you might not be the person to deliver my baby?" I asked.

"Might not. And if you go into labor on a day that we're all on vacation, it could be a total stranger delivering your baby." She winked at me. Ordinarily I'd be really upset that this new midwife was already giving me worst-case-scenario jokes. But I actually found her kind of funny.

The next week at Dr. New York's office, Winnie popped into my exam room. "Did you *love* Annie?!"

"She was awesome! I really like her a lot." I considered expanding on what I liked about Annie and why, but instead I told her, "I want to see the baby move today."

"Oh! Okay, well, let's wake that baby up, shall we?" Winnie giggled and jiggled my tummy with her hand. "Wake up, little peanut! We're getting ready to take your picture!"

Dr. New York walked in a few minutes later and shook Phillip's hand before assuming the position at my feet and preparing for the ultrasound. "She wants to see the baby move, Doc," Winnie said.

"Oh yeah? Let's see if we can make that happen." He smiled.

"Isn't it cute how she always wears skirts?" Winnie asked.

The ultrasound machine flashed a picture of my baby on the screen, and within about thirty seconds, I saw it.

Movement.

The little peanut (it actually looked like a little peanut) with hands and feet began to wiggle. It wiggled slowly back and forth, sort of like it was trying to hula-hoop. It stopped wiggling and then began wiggling again several times while I stared in utter, complete, eye-watering amazement.

"There! Wiggles!" Winnie shouted.

"Looking good," Dr. New York said as he measured and clicked.

The entire ultrasound procedure lasted about five minutes. It was the most glorious five minutes I could recall. Better than finding out I was pregnant. Better than hearing the baby's heartbeat. My baby could wiggle! It could do a little baby dance. It was alive and kicking—literally—in my belly.

After seeing this, Phillip and I walked around the house for the next week doing the "Baby Dance." It's slow and mostly involves swaying your hips back and forth with your elbows at your sides with a little smile on your face. Try it.

· · · · · · · · · · · · · · · · · · · ·

I scheduled a massage with a very hippy dippy, spiritual-type guy. Everyone told me I needed a pregnancy massage from this guy. (That's one thing that happens when you get pregnant—friends with kids who have been waiting for you to get pregnant begin to share their secrets.) I couldn't imagine why, but I booked an appointment for a Saturday afternoon.

It was a little bit cold outside (for Florida) so Phillip turned on the heat in the car on the way to drop me off at the masseuse's office. That was the first time I learned how directly correlated my happiness now was to the temperatures surrounding me. The smell of the car heater made me feel ever so sick, and the heat felt a hundred times hotter than any heat had ever felt. I couldn't open my mouth to speak or breathe for the entire twenty-minute drive. I kept my mouth shut and prayed, staring out the window, until I finally tried cracking it and breathing fresh air, which helped only a little.

"Did you mean to just crack the window?" Phillip asked.

"I did," I said without opening my mouth too wide.

"Okay. Well. Do you want me to open more windows?"

I didn't answer until we'd parked and I'd gotten out of the car and puked. "No, I'm fine. I don't like heat now."

The masseuse was about six four and looked to be in his late fifties. He had gray hairs in his beard and bright blue eyes. This was not the person I was expecting. But all of his spiritual woo-woo toys around the tiny lavender room were right up my alley, so I ate up all of his "Let your body breathe" and "Love your baby and your body" comments as he began to work on my feet.

As he sat across from me after the massage, his eye twinkled. He told me that my baby was very healthy, and I was going to experience a beautiful pregnancy. I immediately called Phillip and told him we had nothing to worry about because the hippy dippy massage therapist told me everything was okay. There was just something about him that made me think he knew what he was talking about.

CHAPTER 16

The Highs and the Lows

Eating was getting even more interesting in week nine, but it felt so good that our lives didn't have to be feel as limited anymore. During one lunch, I ate an entire pastrami on rye sandwich. I can't explain this, because the thought of hot, sliced sandwich meat has always made me gag. But something about that warm, spiced beef, or pork, or ... wait, what *is* pastrami? Anyway, I covered it in mustard and ate the whole thing. As well as the onion rings.

At another meal, I drank a huge glass of lemonade, ate only the colorful vegetables out of my salad, and ordered clam linguine. Yes, I said clam linguine. I don't know what I was thinking, but I liked it that night. The next day, the leftovers made me want to petition the government to have clams banned from the United States.

Liking weird food one day and hating it the next day became a pattern my poor husband finally got used to. Whereas food during my attempts to get pregnant was strictly limited to a few things approved by my doctor, food during my pregnancy was strictly limited to a few things approved by my body. One day I wanted to eat broccoli forever, and the next day the mere thought of broccoli made me dry heave and then reach for the cherry pie filling. Some days I loved spaghetti sauce straight from the jar and other days I needed ripe cucumbers. Elbow macaroni, whole cantaloupes, kale, olives, and orange juice all made the rounds.

There was no pattern to the foods my body craved, and while it felt good to be away from the infertility diet, it felt weird to hate foods that

I normally loved, like grilled chicken or orange juice (because after a few glasses of orange juice, I suddenly hated *it* too). I wasn't vomiting or experiencing diarrhea too much by week ten. My body just developed hundreds of little on/off lights on a giant switchboard in my stomach, installed a bunch of shorted-out wires, and then watched to see which weird combination would light up next.

On a drive home from my favorite sushi restaurant (where I ate only cooked sushi because eating raw sushi meant sudden death according to The Google), I suddenly got the sniffles. I sniffled again and again. I finally reached up, touched under my nose, and then looked at my fingers. Blood.

"Um, Phil? Do you have a napkin or paper towel or something?"

"I think there are some tissues in the glove box," Phillip responded. "Why?"

"I have a nosebleed."

"What? Why?" he asked, scrambling for the tissues. "Are you sick?"

"No. I'm pregnant."

"Pregnant people get nosebleeds?"

"I think so," I said, holding my head up and stuffing the tissue into my nostril. "I think I read that somewhere."

It wasn't a bad nosebleed, and it stopped by the time we got home, but I felt dizzy and overall yucky. The only other nosebleed I'd had was in fourth grade, so this was weird.

When we got home, I stood in front of our full-length mirror. I was wearing a pair of "fat-day" khakis and a billowy top as I tipped my head back to continue catching the blood. I moaned. "Look at this. These khakis are already too tight."

"You're pregnant, Erin," Phillip said.

"I look all bloated and disgusting after I eat now."

"You look like a normal woman, Erin."

"Bleah. I feel like a big marshmallow."

"You look fine, Erin. Do you want some spaghetti sauce?"

"No, thank you. I hate spaghetti sauce. I mean, I hate it today."

The next day I stood up from the couch and felt a pain in my lower abdomen so incredible that I was pretty sure either my appendix had ruptured or my baby was The Incredible Hulk. I didn't want to alarm

Phillip, who was still sitting on the couch, so I did the "Ooo!" noise and tried to hide my winces by looking out the window. For a split second, I thought I was in deep trouble. And then the pain went away. *Oookay*, I thought. *Don't google this.*

And I didn't. I decided I would ask Dr. New York at my final appointment. (Score? Erin: 1. Google: Well, who cares how many points Google had?)

One morning in my tenth week, I woke up, ate a little something, and started working on my computer. Suddenly, I came to a dramatic realization.

I didn't feel sick!

Could it be over this quickly? Could I have dodged the sick-until-sixteen-weeks bullet? It didn't seem fair after all I had been through that I suddenly felt fine. I almost felt guilty. Maybe *real* moms felt sick longer, and I was just getting away with something?

While the nausea was all but gone, other symptoms started creeping in. I've never been a girl people thought of as "flat." It's not that I'm a Dolly Parton lookalike, but there were many pictures in college taken by males at BBQs and beach days that somehow didn't manage to include my head. So, when I put on my bra one morning and it *no longer fit*, I had a mild panic attack. How big could this baby be that it needed another size's worth of milk already? I walked into the kitchen that morning in a tank top and shorts, and Phillip did a double take before saying something along the lines of, "Holy crap, woman."

I decided perhaps it was time to visit the bra section of Target. And perhaps the sweater section as well.

• •

Our ten-week appointment was bittersweet. It was our last appointment before transitioning to the regular ob-gyn and my midwife, Annie. The wonderful nurses and doctors began saying their good-byes almost the moment we walked in the door. Everyone was a little teary. I had been at this office once, sometimes twice, sometimes even three times every week for the past year! These people—Dr. New York, Pam, Winnie, Sally the Shot Nurse—had become like family, helping us to grow our own family.

They gave us the big ultrasound room so that everyone could come in and see how our baby was growing. Pam, Winnie, Sally, and Dr. New York all crowded around me as we watched the screen.

"Look at my baby!" I screeched. Someone pointed out how long the baby's legs looked. Someone else touched the screen to show where the umbilical cord was beginning to form. We all ooooed and ahhhed at the baby's fingers and toes and crazy little movements. It was one of the best days I can remember.

When "my" nurses, doctors, and friends all left the room, only Winnie was left. She went over a few last things with me, including coming off pelvic rest (Yay! I could salsa dance if I wanted!) and continuing to eat as cleanly as possible given my body's issues with sugar. As she hugged Phillip and me good-bye, she stopped. "Do you hear that music?"

We both listened and realized it was coming from the behind the door of the connecting room. "Yeah," I said. "Country Western?"

"That's where we keep the eggs for in-vitro fertilization. They're in little refrigerators in there. Our lab technician believes the eggs do better when they get to listen to music!"

I smiled. "A bunch of little cowboys and cowgirls are about to be born!"

We did a fun little two-step shimmy before Winnie left.

Oh, how I would miss these people.

On my way out, I remembered that shooting pain I had felt in my stomach the previous week. I grabbed a nurse in the hallway, one I didn't really know, and asked her about it. She had wild curly hair and a face that had often smiled at me in the halls. In a very southern accent, she shouted, "Ooohwa! Yoo mean shewters?"

I just looked at her.

"Like, shootin' pains, riiight?"

"Yeah, right in my belly."

"Yep. Those're shewters! It's just yer tendons stretchin' to fit the baby in there! I had 'em, too! Totally normal."

Shooters. Cute name for a horrible, paralyzing pain.

With questions answered and my last beautiful baby video at the reproductive office recorded, we paid our final bill. Most of the nurses and doctors were up front near billing and they hummed the graduation song as Phillip and I walked down the hall and out of the office. We smiled at each other and made it almost all the way to the car before I doubled over in pain.

"Shooter?"

I grimaced. "Yep."

• •

People kept using the term "baby brain" around me.

"Did you get the baby brain yet?"

"You know, that baby brain doesn't go away when the baby is born."

I'd never heard of it before being pregnant. What the heck was baby brain? Just an excuse mothers use when they forget things?

During my eleventh week, we were packing for a trip we were taking to see my mom the next morning (a short, three-hour drive south), I walked out into the living room from the bedroom to a scene out of *Backdraft*. I shouted an expletive and Phillip, startled, shouted, "*What!*" from the bedroom.

"*I don't know!*" I shouted back.

The entire living room was filled with dark brown smoke. I knew Phillip was in the bedroom, so I didn't have to worry that he'd spontaneously combusted the way he had in that dream I'd had a few weeks prior. The house was just burning down. That's all.

I started hunting for the culprit, and after a few seconds, I made my way into the kitchen.

"Erin, what happened? What's going on?" Phillip shouted from the bedroom doorway.

The smoke detectors were screaming at the top of their lungs as if, well, as if the house was on fire. The dogs were barking. It was loud and confusing, and I didn't know what was going on until I remembered the popcorn.

A short while earlier, I had decided to make some popcorn. We make the stove-top kind—buy the kernels, put oil in the pan, and shake it all together over heat until it pops. My mom always used to make it that way, and when Phillip and I moved in together, he started making it that way too.

"Erin! Oh, *geez!*" Phillip sang as he opened up every window and door in the house.

That's right. I had put two tablespoons of oil and two tablespoons of corn kernels on the stove to make popcorn and then simply walked away to pack for our trip. Somewhere in my brain, I just sort of assumed the automated kitchen feature I had asked for but didn't get when we bought our house had been installed after dinner and before our late-night snack.

"I'm sorry!" I repeated over and over again. It took about an hour and a half for the smoke to drain out of the main rooms and another week before the house no longer smelled like burnt popcorn. (And if you've never smelled a house that smells like burnt popcorn, you're really missing out on a special treat. *Especially* if you're pregnant.) And, to boot, I'd ruined a perfectly good pot. It was the oatmeal pot. Now what would we make oatmeal in?

I went to bed that night in my smoke-filled sheets with an empty tummy and a hurumphy husband. As I drifted off to sleepland, it suddenly occurred to me … *Oooooh.* That's baby brain.

• • • • • • • • • • • • • • • • • • •

I was twelve weeks pregnant. After spending a few days with my mom, enjoying the beach and the sunshine and a few well-cooked meals, we packed up our stuff and began our good-byes. Just then, I felt that irritating feeling in my nose. Another nosebleed.

Twelve weeks is when you're out of the quote/unquote "danger zone." Miscarriage is far less common after twelve weeks. This felt amazing. I knew consciously that pregnancy complications could arise at any point. *Any.* But I also knew that, beyond twelve weeks, the percentage of pregnancy problems goes way down. This one little milestone meant that I could take a deep breath and begin—just begin—to let it out. I worried a tiny bit less each and every morning.

By this point, I was almost back to my normal self when an interesting characteristic began to make itself known. It happened one day when I was putting on my jeans. It was just a little bit extra of "me" around my middle. It wasn't enough to make me look pregnant. It was juuuust enough to look fat. The kind of fat that someone looks at and says, "Well, come on, she could do something about that. Lay off the Oreos and ramen noodles, lady."

I also started having more and more trouble sleeping. Not because of the constant peeing on account of my new hormones, but because of the constant anticipation of the peeing. I'd wake up over and over again wondering, *Is this the time I finally have to give in to the pee I feel building up in my bladder? And if I do, should I try to keep my eyes closed the entire time, or just succumb to the pee and walk into the bathroom upright with my eyes open?*

One more thing. Cramps. Foot cramps, to be exact. I'd experienced five, maybe six real cramps in my lifetime. I'd never been a cramper. But now, suddenly, the second I put my feet up or lay down in bed, I would get a foot cramp so bad that I had to wiggle back and forth like a big, juicy earthworm on a hot sidewalk. My mom suggested eating mustard and putting a bar of soap in my sheets to quell the foot cramps. I laughed at her ridiculous ideas and immediately employed both of them. Don't tell her, but they totally worked.

● ● ● ● ● ● ● ● ● ● ●
CHAPTER 17
● ● ● ● ● ● ● ● ● ● ●

I Just Want to Feel Normal

Our first real visit with Annie was interesting. She started with a jokey "Still pregnant?"

"Yep!" I said back, even thought I was thinking, *Why? Did you think I wouldn't be? Did you see something the first time we spoke that made you think I might not still be pregnant? Is it my posture? I should be sitting up straighter. I need to go see the chiropractor.*

Annie explained we would do a basic history, a pelvic exam (hey, at least it's not pelvic *rest*), and then she would perform a first trimester screen. And, because I was automatically qualified as being a "high risk pregnancy" because of my infertility treatments, I also had to make an appointment to see a high-risk doctor who didn't know me or anything about my pregnancy.

So I was really looking forward to *that*.

The high-risk doctor was in a different practice altogether, one that was dedicated to complicated pregnancies. Even though everything about my pregnancy so far seemed normal, it was an extra precautionary step to ensure we weren't missing anything. And if Annie suggested it, I was on board.

Annie also suggested a visit to get to know the other doctor in the practice in case I ended up having a C-section. Annie didn't perform C-sections as a midwife, but she did everything else.

The ob-gyn's name is ... well, I called him Old Man Winter—aka OMW. He had been an ob-gyn for what appeared to be three hundred years. Ob-gyns are the medical brains. They are there to do the surgeries, handle any complications during pregnancy, and they typically recommend more medical intervention than a midwife. A midwife, on the other hand, is usually more comfortable with letting the body do its thing.

But Annie—Annie was a nice combination of the two. She made it very clear to me from the beginning that any of my choices were acceptable to her and that a baby would come out of me no matter what.

OMW joined us in the exam room just prior to the pelvic exam, and with the two of them cornered, I asked every question I could think of, most of which involved whether or not I could dye my hair or use my regular face wash. You know, the important things. They asked if I was exercising and how much, what I was eating, and if I'd had any alcohol. They suggested things like not eating sushi or soft cheeses or lunch meats or sprouts. Seeing as how I had Google HQ on speed dial, I already knew not to eat these things, but it had never occurred to me to ask Google *why* I shouldn't eat these things. Annie explained to me that being pregnant didn't automatically make me allergic to those foods. It was because, if I was the unfortunate recipient of any bacteria, such as *Listeria* or *E. coli*, I now I had a child growing inside of me that would also be susceptible to any of the repercussions.

Annie performed most of the question parade while OMW basically just shook my hand and read through my charts. He was nice enough but didn't really participate, except I do think he asked me something about nausea or baseball or something. Whatever.

"Okay, I'm just going to have you lie down and relax." Annie pulled out a small machine. "I'm going to rub this little wand over your belly and see if we can find the baby's heartbeat." She put a little bit of jelly on my stomach and gently rubbed it with the wand while a radio transmitter crackled. The whole thing reminded me of the movie *Contact* wherein Jodie Foster listened for life on another planet. The machine made scratchy noises, and gurgly noises, and I looked at Annie anxiously to see if I was actually hearing something I should be hearing. Finally, the scratchy noises synced up and became rhythmic. Before I could even squeal with excitement, Annie said, "There it is! Found it! That was fast! Baby sounds strong!"

Our baby's heartbeat.

Phillip and I looked at each other with huge, shit-eating grins, like two people who had never heard a heartbeat before. Yes, we'd heard it on the internal ultrasounds in Dr. New York's office, but never like this. This felt real, like what other *normal* women who get pregnant the *normal* way hear. No fancy machines. Just a little Doppler effect and my baby making heartbeat noises. I was euphoric. And on top of it all, Annie said it had been easy to find. That made me feel as if I was doing something really right, despite the fact that I literally had no control over how easy it was to find my baby's heartbeat.

As we left, we made our appointment with the high-risk doctor via the receptionist. She called, relayed their schedule to us, and we chose a time the very next week to get it over with.

Everyone said that, once I got pregnant, no matter how many interventions I needed, I wouldn't even remember the struggle. And they were half right. Once I got pregnant, I didn't spend time dwelling on the fact that I hadn't been able to get pregnant naturally, but no one seemed to want to let me forget it either—ten weeks of infertility ultrasounds and now a high-risk OB appointment to further investigate my pregnancy. I didn't want to be ungrateful, but I also wished I could feel *normal* at some point.

Phillip and I went to the high-risk appointment the next day. I sat in a lobby *full* of women. Older women, younger women, women with kids, women by themselves, sick women, healthy women. All of us were in the same boat, waiting to ride out the waves of a high-risk pregnancy. I wanted to talk to them. *Why are you in for?* I would ask, and then commiserate about how silly this all was. But I didn't. I just sat and read through an old magazine and tried not to touch the parts of it that were sticky.

"Erin Salem?"

"Yes!" I stood up with Phillip, and we walked to the oddly-placed door in the middle of the room. I wasn't showing very much of a baby belly at this point, and I wanted so badly to waddle like a big pregnant woman. I was so jealous of that waddle. A nurse weighed me without really talking to me and then pulled out a finger pricker to take some of my blood. When I asked what the blood sample was for, she explained that the high-risk doctor required that I take a new, state-of-the-art blood test. It checks for Down syndrome, Trisomy 21, and Trisomy 18. These are all chromosomal abnormalities that are more often present in pregnancies that result from fertility treatments. The test also looks for other abnormalities such as cardiac disorders. It is becoming more common because it can identify risks months sooner than the old Alpha-fetoprotein (AFP) tests that were conducted in the second trimester. (I don't completely understand what those last three sentences mean, so you should probably google them.) I would get the results by the end of my appointment.

Once she'd taken my blood, she led me into an ultrasound room.

"We're doing an ultrasound?" I asked with excitement. Phillip had a big grin on his face, already getting his camera out of my purse, which we'd put in there just in case.

"Yes, we need to check the baby's spinal growth and cranial ..." I stopped listening. *I get to see my baby!* I practically catapulted onto the exam table. This time, she got to use the jelly on my belly and the regular ultrasound machine like the ones you see on TV. No more internal ultrasounds for me! Wow! This was a step toward normal!

The nurse wrote things down without talking to me, clicked buttons on her machines, and finally turned around with the belly jelly in her hand. "Okay, go ahead and lie back," she said. I wanted to say, "Okay, sounds great. I'm Erin, by the way. This is Phillip. This is our first pregnancy. We are really excited. Thanks for asking." But my animosity all went away when, within seconds, a flash on the screen was a perfect, real-looking baby. A baby-looking baby. It had long arms and long legs, a body, a head. And it was moving and wiggling! And then, the baby jumped. No, it didn't roll over or stretch. It *jumped*. "Did it just *jump*?" I screeched.

"Oh, um. I think so. I need to get this measurement here." It was as if the woman was brain dead—all except for the parts of her brain that took measurements and notes.

Then the baby jumped again.

"My baby is jumping! It jumps! I don't even feel that!"

"Wow!" Phillip exclaimed. "That's amazing!"

Without telling us, the woman then switched the ultrasound machine to a four-dimension ultrasound, so we suddenly had no idea what we were looking at except that maybe everything in my body had just spontaneously turned into marshmallows.

"That's the face right there," she said dryly, "but it's not really too clear." And she was right. I could kind of see what looked like a face, or maybe a muddy puddle, I didn't know. I couldn't figure out where the baby stopped and where I began. Phillip and I both stared at the screen tilting our heads in opposite directions until the nurse turned the machine off. "All set. Now we'll have to wait for the blood work results, and you can be on your way."

"Oh. Okay," I said. "Did you happen to see any genitalia? I know it's early, but I was just wondering." The nurse sighed. She begrudgingly turned the machine back on, as if at some point a doctor had told her that she needed to try to be nicer to patients, and so now she was "trying." She fiddled around with the ultrasound wand until the baby was back in view.

"The leg is in the way," she said, moving the wand around. "I can't see. That could be labia there, though."

Phillip and I both chuckled. Hehe. Labia.

"But I really can't tell …" As she trailed off, a tall doctor walked in. "How are we dooooing?" he asked.

"Fine," I answered, immediately realizing he probably wasn't asking me.

"All the measurements are here, 4-Ds are here," the nurse answered before walking out of the room.

"Nice to meet you," I said to the nurse quietly.

"Okay, it looks like we have a beautiful baby, here," Tall Doctor said. "I'll just look through these pictures and send you on your way." He clicked through the pictures on the screen, nodding and saying, "Mmhmm, mmhmm," and writing down a few more notes. "Okeeey! All set, baby looks good. Nice to meet you both."

"Nice to meet you," I said quietly again.

After he'd left, Phillip and I rolled our eyes at each other. This was such a different experience from our appointments with Dr. New York or our few visits with Annie. We both felt so lucky that we would be in kinder hands throughout the rest of the pregnancy. Not to mention we'd be working with doctors who knew our names. Or asked our names.

While we waited for my blood work, Phillip and I couldn't ignore the possibility that something *could* be wrong with our baby and we were moments from finding out.

"What will we do if our baby has Down syndrome?" he asked.

"We'll have it, and I think we'll probably be really good at raising it," I answered.

"If it's one of the disorders where they only live a few months, should we have the baby then?"

"I say yes. I mean, if that's what we're supposed to get, then it will probably be an amazing learning experience. Don't you think?"

"Yeah. I agree. And I mean, a heart condition or some other congenital abnormality seems unlikely, right?"

"I think so. I don't have any of that in my family. Of course, I didn't think I had diabetes in my family and it turns out I'm prediabetic, so …"

"Well, either way, we're having the baby, right?"

We paused. We both thought about it. I couldn't imagine not having this baby. And I wouldn't think that Phillip would consider terminating the pregnancy an option under any circumstances. Unless, of course, my life was at risk. But suddenly this conversation felt heavy, scary, and like maybe we should have talked about this before now.

"Right. We're having it either way," I finally answered.

Fifteen minutes later, results were in. Our test results were all normal. I couldn't help but feel heavy for a few days, wondering what it must feel like to get results that changed everything. I silently sympathized with those women.

After the "high-risk" appointment was over, I wouldn't have another ultrasound for four weeks. Four weeks. How would I even know if I was still pregnant in four weeks?

While lamenting about waiting more than a month to have another ultrasound (when most women only had two to three for their *entire* pregnancies!), I got my next BabyProgress email. For thousands of years, women had given birth without knowing the gender of their baby until the baby popped out. I could make it four weeks. This email recommended that I rent a fetal heart monitor online. I thought about it but decided that this would just be giving in to my fears, and also to BabyProgress's affiliate marketing program.

One day, I leashed up Charlie and Bella for our daily walk adventure and, at the end of the driveway, I decided to walk them to the right instead of the left. They were immediately a little confused but so thrilled to be on a walk (because they hadn't walked on leashes in nearly twenty-four hours) that they didn't care.

My neighborhood was quaint and full of older homes and older people. The trees that line the street were old, too, and bushy with green leaves. Everyone's little lawns were very well manicured with brightly colored flowers near all the front doors.

We made it about twenty yards before a truck started pulling out of a driveway a few doors down. I stopped and waited, and a man got out to manually close his garage. Based on Charlie's reaction, I can only assume he had once been attacked by a garage. He ran behind me so fast that it spooked Bella, who quickly followed him. Their two leashes wrapped perfectly around my ankles in a criss-cross, yanked my arms behind me (because the leashes were attached to my wrists), and swept my legs out and away while I splatted face first onto—you guessed it—my stomach (and chest and face).

I immediately whipped around to see that both dogs were still attached to me. And in the next breath I said to myself, "Oh crap! I'm pregnant and I just landed on my stomach." The idiot who was standing less than ten feet from me shouted "Ya'lright?" from the garage. He never even offered me a hand. I slowly got myself up and walked home with leash-burned wrists, sore knees, and a questionable feeling in my stomach.

After much deliberation (Am I "That Girl" if I call a doctor? Will I look back and regret it if I don't?), I finally decided to call my doctor. The office was closed by the time I made the call, which meant that I would have to speak with an on-call doctor. I left a message with the on-call service and waited by the phone.

About ten minutes later, James Earl Jones called. I'm not positive it was him, and I never knew he was a doctor, but I spoke with a man whose voice was so deep it made my crystal glasses rattle. He assured me I was probably fine but that I should call my doctor on Monday to schedule an appointment. Wow. Talk about What-If Monsters all weekend long.

On Monday, the nurse at my doctor's office assured me that I was fine but offered me an appointment to come in and listen to the baby's heartbeat to be sure. I thought for a second and politely declined. I hung up and immediately ordered a rental fetal heart monitor from my BabyProgress email, which shipped in twenty-four hours for free. When it arrived, I walked straight into my room and listened to the little peanut's heart beating away.

The rental fetal heart monitor: the control freak's ultimate pregnancy weapon.

CHAPTER 18

Getting my Mom Card

I was feeling good enough to exercise again so I signed up for five classes of prenatal yoga. I had done some yoga and Pilates before I ever tried getting pregnant. I knew I wanted to feel like one of those active pregnant women.

I walked into the first class and was *clearly* the earliest pregnancy in the room. The room itself was about the size of a bedroom with mats and blankets strewn about. Tapestries hung from three of the walls, and the fourth one was mirrored. All these big, beautiful, round bellies on their yoga mats made me feel almost inadequate! Really? Isn't *anyone* in her first trimester?

The instructor walked in. She was one of those pregnant women who pregnant women love to hate: tiny body, pretty little legs, strong but slender arms, beautiful hair, perfect boobs, and a pregnant belly that only gathered into a teeny, tight ball in the front of her abdomen. I looked at myself in the mirror. A little fat, thighs a little wide, absolutely no waist. So far, prenatal yoga was not making me feel like a beautiful pregnant girl.

The class started with everyone announcing her month and a miracle that had happened that week.

"Well, I'm twenty-four weeks, and the baby flipped over in my belly this week!" said one.

"I'm thirty-two weeks, and I learned that our little boy is just the right size for his age," another cooed.

When it was my turn, I said, "I'm thirteen weeks, and this week I didn't feel like barfing every time I smelled dish soap."

It didn't get the laugh you would expect.

The class consisted of pretty typical yoga moves. That is, until we started rocking our babies. Yeah. We rocked them. In our bellies. But that's cute, right? You'd go along with that.

Then we started singing to our babies. Out loud. Singing about what beautiful rays of light the babies were. *Hmph*, I thought. There was so much estrogen in that room it was suffocating. I'm all for hippy dippy, but even I was feeling this was a little much. Then we were instructed to speak, out loud, to our babies, thanking them for choosing us to be their mothers. I followed directions, all the while thinking, "I know you chose me because you think this is all just as over-the-top as I do."

As soon as the class was over, I went to the grocery store and bought five cans of ravioli (because they were on sale, five for $10).

Begrudgingly, I went to the second class a few days later because I'd already paid for it. I thought, if just *one* woman would walk in looking less than round and beautiful, I might feel better. I realized this was completely egotistical, but if I was going to sing to my baby that people couldn't even tell was there, I wanted someone else to look stupid too. Finally, a tall woman walked in just as the door closed. She looked like me: a little bit pregnant but mostly like she'd eaten a big piece of cake. I silently rejoiced. As we went around the room announcing our month and miracle, I contemplated sharing the joy of ravioli in a can but instead chose something about how amazing our baby's heartbeat is. I also loudly proclaimed my month. "I'm almost fourteen weeks!" I think I said it right to the other woman, who looked at me and smiled. Oh, we are connecting. We totally get each other here. She felt fat. I felt fat. I waited for it to be her turn and for her to say something like, "I'm thirteen weeks and I just feel fat." And then I would stand up and high five her and shout, "You go girl!"

Then, of course, she stood up and said, "Hi, I'm Mindy and I'm twenty-six weeks."

Yep. Mindy was more than halfway through her pregnancy and she barely looked pregnant. Awesome. Prenatal yoga just got better and better.

After we rocked and sang to and thanked our babies, I went home and ate more ravioli. I called the next week before the class was to resume and told them I had a conflict. Ravioli conflict.

My pants were tight now and I was using a Belly Band. This is a giant hair band that you pull up over the top of your pants because you can't button them anymore but you haven't bought maternity pants yet. Not until my seventeenth week did *other* people start noticing my belly. Suddenly people were patting and rubbing my little tum-tum! And I was so excited! This was the dream! It was the one time in my life that touching my fat belly didn't make me feel fat. I'd fantasized about being the pregnant belly in the room everyone wanted to rub. It was every bit as good as I imagined it would be. I felt so proud and not fat.

One day, I was walking through the grocery store with Phillip when I suddenly thought of something else I wanted, and Phillip jaunted off to find it. While I looked through the millions of different kinds of soup, I overheard a conversation between a mom and her daughter.

"Mom, are you going to buy that here?"

"Yeah. Why?"

"Well, you know, I'll bet if you go to Walmart you could get it cheaper."

I chuckled out loud, thinking how cute it was that the woman's daughter was so cost conscious. I must have chuckled out louder than I thought, because the mom laughed and put her hand on my shoulder as she walked by. I turned around and smiled at her. She said, "You know what? You're right to acknowledge that with a chuckle! My kid pays attention to prices, and that is pretty cool! High-five!" She high-fived her daughter. I smiled, thinking about how cool that moment must have been for that mom. And then she dropped the bomb. She turned back, smiled at me, pointed at my belly, and said, "I love that I shared that with a fellow mom!"

Fellow mom? Holy crap, I'm a fellow mom! Did anyone hear that? And that mom can *tell* I'm a fellow mom! That was a moment I will never forget. Week fifteen, and it looked as if I might have joined the club. Mom Club!

One thing that amazed me about being pregnant and starting to "show" was how much people wanted to talk about it. A pregnant woman is either an anomaly or a fellow club member. Women loved to ask me how far along I was or when I was due.

(Men, though, didn't talk about my bump. They opened doors for me instead or allowed me to do things first that really weren't necessary, like choosing my apples from the produce stand or taking a menu at a restaurant counter. Men seemed mostly concerned that I get from place to place safely and have constant access to food. I guess it's an instinct?)

But there are always the women with an opinion. These are the ones you have to watch out for. In line at the grocery store that same day, a girl in front of me chatted with the friend who was with her in line about how she gave up full-sugar Mountain Dew and switched to diet because she was breastfeeding. Was I going to judge her? Nope. I judged pregnant women for eating Chef Boyardee until I got pregnant and ate four cans a week (okay, seven). I no longer judged any of them. But then the checker lady had to have an opinion. She ran the Diet Mountain Dew across the laser beep and said, "Well, I don't think you're supposed to drink caffeine when you're pregnant or breastfeeding." The breastfeeding mother laughed it off, obviously having dealt with The Opinion before. "Yeah, they say a lot of things. My kids are all fine."

"Well," The Opinion went on, "you don't know right away, right?"

Breastfeeding Mom again ignored the obviously wide-open door to take The Opinion down and shrugged. I, being a new member of the club, felt the need to step in. (Also, I tend to step in at inappropriate times.) "I'm pregnant, and I have some form of caffeine every day," I said. "My baby's doing fine."

Breastfeeding Mom looked back at me and smiled. "I'm pretty sure I had a beer or two as well!" She laughed and walked off.

That's right, girl! I thought it. I didn't say it. Now it was just me and The Opinion. "My friend is pregnant, and she told me she can't have any caffeine and absolutely no alcohol," The Opinion announced.

I puffed up. "There are a lot of opinions and a lot of data, but fortunately for us, we all get to make choices for ourselves."

The Opinion shook her head. "I just can't see putting my baby at risk."

Luckily for her, she was bagging my groceries when she said that, and the transaction was over, leaving me without enough time to shove my ramen noodles down her throat. So, I looked The Opinion square in the eyes and said, "You know, as I said, it's up to each of us individually. But I can assure you, somewhere in Italy right now, there is a pregnant woman eating a delicious piece of unpasteurized cheese with her glass of wine."

As I walked away, I felt confident. Maybe for the first time in my life, I felt confident to say what I thought without worrying about what others thought. Pregnancy gave me confidence, a sheath of "I don't care" wrapped around me. I was ready to do only what was best for me and my baby. I really wanted this confidence to last. I wanted to move into motherhood keeping what I'd learned so far in this process tightly packaged in my pocket like a cheat sheet. I loved this feeling.

I made it all the way outside before I realized I'd left Phillip in the store, and I was too afraid to walk back inside after my grand, confident exit.

The irony isn't lost on me.

CHAPTER 19

The Big Reveal

Between my boobs growing to the size of melons and my stomach expanding *straight* out in front of me, my lower back was starting to bend under the pressure. On some mornings, I woke up and couldn't stand up straight for several minutes while I whined and bumped into walls trying to get to the bathroom.

I also continued to get nosebleeds. While some were just a few drops, others were gushers like the ones I'd had at my mom's. I started carrying paper towels with me. I could sneeze and get a nosebleed, cough and get a nosebleed; hell, I could smile and get a nosebleed. My ob-gyn did finally call me to explain that pregnancy nosebleeds are very common and to try not to worry about anything but wearing white shirts. I didn't have another appointment with Annie until our twenty-week gender ultrasound, so I decided to try to wait it out.

And, of course, I was eagerly anticipating that twenty-week gender ultrasound. What *was* I having? I was still a month away from my appointment so, to find out, I consulted a gender prediction test. Have you seen these? They're ridiculous. You can't possibly think they're real—a small cup with "magic crystals" inside that change color when combined with urine to determine the sex of your baby. Dumb. And certainly not accurate enough to spend forty dollars on at the drug store. I mean, it's literally a pee-in-a-cup test to determine the genetic makeup of your baby. *Pah-lease.*

So, anyway, I bought one.

The next morning, I rolled out of bed and went straight to the bathroom to deposit my urine onto the magical crystals. Orange meant girl and green meant boy. I got the camera ready and told Phillip to stand by as I was about to announce to him whether he was having a son or a daughter. The crystals immediately made the urine change color. I took a picture. I mean, it was pretty clear. The crumbly little crystals sitting in the bottom of the cup turned my pee orange. Orange meant girl! We were having a girl!

We danced around and giggled and shouted, "Baby girl!" Phillip took about twenty pictures. We went into the kitchen to grab cups of coffee (Yes, The Opinion, I had caffeine!), and returned to the bathroom a few minutes later to giggle some more. That was when we saw this: Orange pee with green spots.

It was then that I decided to actually read the directions, because that's how I roll. "Wait ten minutes before you read the results." It had been approximately ten minutes by this point, and the results were much less clear than when I first peed in the cup. Now it was sort of half boy, half girl.

Holy shit. Half boy, half girl? That's like a mother's worst nightmare! Would I have to be one of those women who is forced to *choose* the sex of her baby because s/he came out with both sets? I knew that, inevitably, I'd choose the wrong gender, and my child would grow up resenting me and wanting to be the other sex. What if my baby ended up in a drag show in New York with a name like Mango Scrumptious?

Come to think of it, a son/daughter drag queen/king named Mango Scrumptious sounds amazing. And I love New York. I got kind of excited about it for a second ...

Okay, refocus. Deep breaths. Maybe the test malfunctioned. Maybe I got bad crystals. Or maybe it had been right in the first place—girl—and then slowly changed color because of an environmental change like the AC kicking on.

Maybe you shouldn't buy gender predictor tests from the drug store.

When I shared that debacle with my sister-in-law Sharon over the phone later that morning, she asked me, "Have you tried the Chinese gender prediction calendar?"

"Um, no."

"It's really accurate. I have no idea why it works, but it does. Just google it."

So I went into the office, typed in "Chinese gender predictor," and hit enter. And that's when 1,960,000 results popped up (which makes it *even more* credible, right?). They were all different layouts and formats of a Chinese gender predictor. No two the same, but all asking the same two questions: What is your date of conception? and What is your due date?

"How do I know my date of conception?" I asked Sharon.

"What day were you inseminated?" she asked.

"December 17, but that doesn't mean that's the day I got pregnant."

"Yeah. You're right," she said, pausing to think.

"Oh, wait!" I said. "This one says if you don't know your date of conception, it will calculate it for you." This thing was gaining more and more credibility by the second. "I'll just enter in my due date, September 10."

"Yeah. That's fine. That should work," Sharon said, as if we were mechanics trying to find the right screw to keep the engine from falling out of a car.

"Okay. Entered and …" We waited as the little star on the screen spun around, searching for the gender of my baby. "Oh! A girl! I'm having a girl!"

It was quiet for a few seconds.

"Awww! That's awesome!"

We both mildly celebrated.

"Wait. Are you home?" I asked Sharon.

"Yeah."

"You do one. See what yours says for me."

It was quiet again as I heard her clicking the keys of her computer. "Okay. Waiting," she said. I leaned against the office desk. About ten seconds later, she said, "Hmmm. Boy."

"Did you put in the same dates?"

"Yeah. Hmm. Weird."

Except not weird, right? Because we were *relying on a Chinese gender predictor on the internet.*

I hung up with Sharon and called Phillip and told him to do it.

"And just put in the due date?" he asked.

"Yeah."

"Okay. Aaaand … girl. It says girl," he said, placing absolutely no gravity on the results.

"Girl?" I repeated, nodding. "Okay, I got girl, too. And Sharon got boy. So maybe it only works with the parents. I mean, two out of three. So it must be a girl!"

Quiet again.

"Okay, babe. Well, I gotta get back to work."

It really was a red-letter day.

As silly as it sounds (and it *does*), I, for one, was convinced. It wasn't the tests; it was a *feeling*. I was having a girl. And her name was Hazel. Hazel Kate. Phillip wasn't crazy about the name, and my mom straight-up hated it, but I loved it. It came from my favorite band, Sister Hazel. The name of their band had been inspired by a nun, Hazel, who did nonprofit work in Gainesville, Florida, where they're from. I'd been listening to them since I was twelve, and because they never really changed, I never had to change with them, so their songs still took me back to a place of joy. That's why Hazel. Kate was after my mom, Kathleen.

When I imagined Hazel Kate, I imagined lots of snuggling. I saw a sweet little baby whom I held, who wanted to be held by me, and who loved me. But I also had a feeling that, as she grew up, she was going to be a tomboy. I remember my mom and I were on a walk one day, and I told her, "I feel like it is a girl, but she's a kickass girl." I imagined getting her set up in cool-girl activities like woodworking and soccer. I never imagined her being a teacup-and-princess kind of girl. I imagined her always being a little bit dusty, her hair usually not in any kind of order. And I absolutely could not wait to hang out with her.

Finally, when I was nineteen weeks along, we were scheduled for the *real* gender reveal. This ultrasound would measure the baby's head and legs and, without a doubt, there would be a very clear penis or labia to celebrate. (And that is the first time I've ever said that.) That is, barring any major catastrophes like my baby crossing its little legs out of modesty or, worse, having both sets of genitalia as the crystals suggested.

Annie met Phillip and me in the waiting area and motioned for us to come back. "How have you been feeling?" she asked as we walked to the ultrasound room.

"Actually, really good. Some pretty normal cravings and a lot of foot cramps, but in general I feel awesome."

"That's fantastic! I'm just going to feel around on your belly for a few seconds, and then we'll do the ultrasound." She pushed around, seemingly arbitrarily, and then smiled. "Feels good!"

She checked to see if I had any other questions before she left, and since I didn't, I made one up so she'd stay a little longer. "Is my size normal? Have I gained too much weight?"

"You know, you've gained about twenty pounds. We like to see girls gain a total of twenty-eight during pregnancy. At the rate you're growing, you'd be between forty and fifty pounds by the time you deliver. But we just never know if you'll—"

I stopped listening. Shit. I had just been kidding. I had just asked the question because I liked talking to Annie and I didn't like Old Man Winter. Now I was overweight and growing? "Oh. Should I exercise or something?" I asked.

"No. Not really. Maybe walking. But I don't think it's too big of a deal right now. Anything else?"

I looked down. "No," I said.

Old Man Winter had to do the gender ultrasound because he was the doctor, the one with the degree in gender ultrasounding. We waited in the ultrasound room, which was small, but the TV monitor was really big—bigger than the TV we had in our living room! As he walked in, he made a bunch of Old Man Winter jokes. "Ready to find out what color paint to buy? Two legs or three, what do you think? You reckon there'll be a stem on the apple?" His jokes were painful, but we laughed kindly.

He squeezed a *massive* amount of jelly onto my belly, and away we went.

Old Man Winter measured my baby's legs, arms, and head. He showed us the spine and even counted all the fingers and toes. And without warning, he said these words, in this order, "One leg, two legs, and a third leg. That's a baby boy."

Oh. My. God.

"What?" Phillip spun around and smiled at me as if he'd just won a horseracing bet.

My gasp turned to laughter, which turned to tears, which turned into, "A boy?"

"Wow," Phillip said.

"A boy. I have no idea what to do with a boy!" I half laughed, half cried.

"A boy," Phillip repeated.

I stared at my baby's little face. I repeated in my head, Okay. You're a boy. Okay. You're a boy. A boy. That's what you are. A boy! Holy crap …

You're my son.

CHAPTER 20

Halfway There

Our twenty-week ultrasound made me cry, which made my nose bleed.

"Now, you've been having excessive nose bleeds, is that right?" Old Man Winter asked, turning off the ultrasound machine as if my entire life hadn't just changed. Again.

"Yes," I said to the TV screen.

He referred me to an ear, nose, and throat specialist across the hall from him, made a quick call, and sent us right over. I got the sense that they were golfing buddies. Five minutes after finding out we were having a boy, Phillip and I walked across the hall in silence. We didn't care if we were having a boy or a girl. We wanted a baby. We just had really thought it was a girl. And now we had some processing to do!

"Erin?" the receptionist asked.

"Yes."

"Your doctor just called, and we can slide you right into the schedule. Come on back."

Then we sort of forgot all about our big news because the ENT had to open up my nostril with salad tongs, go in and numb the inside of my nose with a needle, and then use a welding tool to cauterize the vein in my nose. It hurt. It smelled like dying skin and burnt hair. And I was having a boy.

On the drive home from the ENT's office, Phillip asked me, "Should we tell our family?"

"Yeah. I guess so. My nose feels weird."

"Who do you want to tell first?" he asked.

"Probably my mom."

"Let's call your mom and then talk to my mom in person tonight. Maybe we'll go over for dinner?" he suggested.

"Yeah. My nose feels sticky inside."

It was all pretty surreal until I finally called my mom later that day. She knew I was going to find out that day, so she answered the phone with glorious anticipation. "Hellooooo?"

"Hi," I said, smiling. "Wanna know what your grandbaby is?"

"Yes!"

"Are you suuuure?"

"Tell me!"

"It's a ..."

"*Tell me!*"

"A baby boy!"

She screamed, cried, giggled—all the normal reactions you'd expect. That's one thing I could always rely on my mom for: great reactions!

A boy. Whoa. As she screamed, I kept remembering I was having a boy!

It's funny the way some women just know what gender baby they're having—a strong feeling or a dream or a premonition. I'd had all of those things. And I felt I should know what the sex of my baby was before he was born because, damnit, I was his mother! He was a part of me! Why hadn't I known the sex of my own baby before now? You hear moms say, "I knew from day one I was having a boy." Well, ladies, I knew from day one I was having a girl. And that girl turned out to have a penis. It made me feel like a jerk. Like I was off balance. My "premonition" was one hundred percent wrong. Not one part of it was right. How could I be so off?

"Well, what's his name?" my mom asked.

His name?

• •

It was right before we moved to Jacksonville. I wasn't pregnant, and we weren't even in the process of not not trying. Phillip and I were in my white Mini Cooper on LA's 405 freeway, driving home in the middle of a sunny afternoon. He drove, and I looked up at the bright blue sky through the sunroof. Phillip was talking about something, and the radio quietly played in the background. It was a normal ride. Then a song came on the radio. A normal song. Not even one that struck me as interesting enough to tell Phillip to stop talking so I could listen. Still, I looked down to see the name of the song on the radio screen: "Abraham."

There are moments in your life when you just know things, when you are clear enough, aligned enough, connected enough to a Universe bigger than what you can see. It's not a voice in your head; it's a feeling that overcomes you and communicates with you in a language you innately understand. It was that moment, in the car, on a normal, sunny day, that I read the name Abraham.

"Abraham. That's our son's name if we have a son," I said out loud, interrupting Phillip.

"Um. Okay," he responded, maybe a little irritated that I was suddenly interrupting him and bringing up babies. "Why?"

"I don't know. That's just what it is. He's Abraham."

"Okay," Phil said.

I didn't push it. I didn't force him to agree. I didn't feel I needed to. I knew what his name was going to be when he arrived. In hindsight, it had been a pretty extraordinary moment in my life. One that taught me that, if I'm quiet and present, I have the ability to know things I'd never considered even wanting to know.

• • • • • • • • • • • • • • • • • • •

On the day we learned that Abe was a boy, I remembered his name on the way home from that ultrasound and visit with the ENT. I looked at the radio display screen, up at the blue sky, and then at Phillip. "Oh my gosh. He's Abraham."

"Whoa. Oh yeah! He is! Right?"

Right.

So when my mom asked me his name, I responded with a feeling of warmth and assurance. "Abraham," I said with a smile.

"Oooooh!" she cooed. "That's beautiful! Honest Abe!" she chortled.

"Abe the babe!" I said back.

• • • • • • • • • • • • • • • • • • •

At one Sunday family dinner with Phillip's parents, they pulled out a bunch of old documents and stories from their family history. My father-in-law, Tommy, is a holocaust survivor, so his history is somewhat well documented. My mother-in-law wanted to see if there was another Abraham somewhere in the family lineage and, if so, what he might have been like. I thought this was so exciting. It was the first time they had taken real interest in this grandchild. With five grandchildren alive and kickin', they'd done the grandchild thing before. The experience was sort of old hat. But now that Abe was an actual person, it felt more as if we were all in this together.

We read stories and biographies of all kinds of interesting characters together until: "Oh, here's one!" my mother-in-law said, delighted. "Uncle Abraham!"

"Really?" I asked, never believing they'd actually find another Abraham.

"Yes! Hmm, let's see ..." She read silently for a few minutes.

I waited patiently. I think she grimaced once. I peered across the table to see if I could read anything. "Well?" I asked, excited and inquisitive.

It turned out the one guy who was named Abraham suffered from depression and was an alcoholic and ended up killing himself. Yay family history!

(So. Just to be clear, Abraham is not named after Uncle Abraham.)

We actually had a wonderful time reading about other, less tragic, members of the family right there at the kitchen table. For a brief moment, I flashed back to a moment almost a year earlier when we had been sitting at that very table. I had felt so out of place then. I hadn't even felt right in my own skin. And now I was belly-laughing and ooing and ahing with *my family*. This was finally beginning to feel like my family.

• • • • • • • • • • • • • • • • • • • •

Phillip and I decided to celebrate that night. We would go on a date. A real date. Just the two of us. Who knew how many of these nights were left?

I had a coupon to The Melting Pot, and since coupons always make food taste better to me, that was our restaurant of choice. It was also the one where we had told Phillip's family we were pregnant, so I thought it might be a cute Throwback Thursday kind of a thing.

If you've ever eaten at The Melting Pot you know that it is possible, nay *almost certain*, that you will overeat at The Melting Pot. You'll eat to the point of, say, hating yourself. We had salads and a vegetable appetizer and a huge meat tray and a chocolate fondue dessert. Every morsel was delicious. I could barely move by the time we were finished, and I momentarily panicked that Phillip might have to roll me to the car.

"Just sit and relax a minute." He smiled at me across the booth being the not-pregnant man that he was.

"You don't have a baby in your belly taking up the space where the food you just ate is supposed to go," I snapped. Phillip, who was unfazed by my snapping, joyfully sat in his food coma.

Eventually, we vacated the table and drove the twenty minutes home while I whined and squirmed about being full of food and full of baby. As soon as we walked in the front door of our house, I bee-lined it to the guest bathroom (which was closer to the front door than our bathroom). I closed the door and sat down, praying for my stomach to release at least some of what I'd just eaten to make some room in my now very maxed-out belly. Nothing was coming, so I picked up a magazine.

I rarely read on the toilet. And I believe reading on the toilet is the cause of all the problems that came next ...

"What?" Phillip asked me as I walked into the living room a few moments later, face made of stone.

"I think ... I think ..."

"What? You think what?" he asked, a tinge panicked. He probably thought my water had broken.

"What does a hemorrhoid feel like?" I asked.

"Do you have one?" he asked.

"*What does it feel like?*" I asked, but it came out like pleading.

"I don't know. It feels like something is coming out. Or hanging around."

"Oh. My. God." I stood there, staring at him, like if I stared long enough, he would tell me it wasn't a hemorrhoid and we could all move on.

"Well. I mean. Touch it. Can you touch it and see if you can feel it?" he asked. I stared at him in blank horror. "Do you want me to look?" Phillip asked.

I started sobbing and ran into the bedroom to throw myself on the bed. Phillip followed.

"Babe? What is wrong?!"

"I touched it, okay? I touched Herman."

"Who is Herman? Your hemorrhoid?"

"Yes, yes, he's my hemorrhoid, and I touched him and I named him and I have a huge belly and an aching back, leg cramps, sore feet, I'm peeing all the time, and now I have a *Herman*. I don't want this. I don't want any of this."

I cried, and Phillip stood still, staring at my drama, probably wondering if he should touch me or keep a healthy distance.

Finally, "It's just a hemorrhoid, Erin ..."

"*Herman*," I interrupted because it made total sense.

"It's just Herman, Erin. And I'm sure it's completely normal to get one in pregnancy. I'm pretty sure we have hemorrhoid cream in the bathroom ..."

"We do?" I asked through my tears.

"Yeah. Don't you remember you saw that segment on the *Today* show about how hemorrhoid cream gets rid of bags under your eyes so you went out and bought some and applied it every day for a month before you realized you've never had bags under your eyes?"

"Oh yeah," I said, sitting up.

"I'll find it for you so you don't have to lean down to look in the cabinets under the sink, and I'll leave it next to the toilet. Okay?" This was a real shining moment for my husband, solving two problems at once.

About twenty minutes later, after I'd mustered up the courage, I sat back down on the toilet next to the Herman antidote. I applied a small amount to my finger and then went ahead a squeezed a much larger amount onto my finger because I immediately decided this was war. I covered Herman in the cream and waited, as if instantly he would shrivel up and disappear.

He did not.

"It says here," Phillip read through the bathroom door, "that as the baby grows and puts pressure on your pelvis, it stretches your anal veins and that can often cause hemorrhoids. Ha! Anal veins." He thought anal veins were funnier than I did.

I went to bed soon thereafter, but every one of the fifteen times I woke up to pee in the middle of the night, I applied more of the Herman antidote. I'm not sure what the maximum usage in a twenty-four-hour period is, but whatever it is, I'm pretty sure I quadrupled it.

I woke up the next morning to shower, and in my "I hate mornings" haze, I'd forgotten about Herman. When he suddenly flashed across my mind like a swift right hook, I closed my eyes and reached. *Please, Lord. Take Herman away.*

Several minutes later I came running (well, walking at a pace faster than the slowest saunter you could possibly imagine) out of the bathroom in a robe screaming, "Babe! It's a miracle! It's a Christmas miracle!"

It was May.

"What?" he shouted.

"Herman is dead!"

"Herman's gone?" he asked, somewhat impressed.

"He's gone and dead and I've killed him!"

He smiled and remarked that this was wonderful news.

I, on the other hand, felt triumphant. I'd killed Herman in *one night* thanks to the cunning overuse of hemorrhoid cream. If anyone had told me on this day at this time that not only would Herman be back, but he would come and go as he pleased forevermore, I would be tempted to spend the rest of my life eating soft foods and fiber-rich smoothies. But no one did, so I celebrated my win.

CHAPTER 21

The Mom Groove

The following week was a normal pregnancy week. I ate entire cantaloupes. I ate ravioli straight from the can. I marveled at how many ways there are to completely avoid bending over. My only struggle was that I couldn't *feel* Abe moving.

Now, I could feel flutters. I could feel weird wriggling sensations. But what I wanted to feel more than anything was a kick. A solid, he's-gonna-be-a-soccer-player kick. With the number of people asking me if they could feel my belly, I was almost embarrassed that I knew they wouldn't feel anything. "Oh, he's sleeping," I'd say when there was no great show. But inside I was thinking, "Please. Please kick right now so I know you have legs and so I feel like a real pregnant girl."

Here I was, twenty-two weeks pregnant, sitting at the kitchen bar eating cottage cheese with cantaloupe on a Wednesday when … it happened. I almost choked. I sat very still and touched a spot just above my belly button where I'd felt it. I breathed slowly and deeply, eyes like pies.

Boop.

I felt it again. A swift, quick, straight-out-of-the-movie-*Alien* sensation. *That had to have been my baby boy's foot.* It felt exactly the way I thought it would feel and still nothing like anything I'd felt before. A tiny, square inch of my belly popped out and then back in. I couldn't believe it! I had a mouth full of cottage cheese just sitting there waiting to be swallowed, and I couldn't move. He did it. He kicked me. And I felt him. And it was the absolute most amazing moment ever.

I sat in that position, cottage cheese in my mouth, finger on the square inch above my belly button for at least five minutes. Eventually I swallowed and refocused on my computer where I took to Facebook to proclaim: "Kick! I just felt my first, real kick!"

Now. Now I was definitely pregnant.

When they tell you it's "so amazing" to feel your baby moving inside of you, there's no way to truly understand it until you feel it. At twenty-three weeks, I woke up constantly at night to change positions, and if I waited a few moments, my baby boy usually changed positions too. He giggled after I ate and stretched while I watched TV. I imagined his movements with the clarity of seeing them on video because the truth was, when he was growing inside me, it didn't feel as if we were separate. It didn't feel as if he were someone I was getting to know. It was that feeling you get when you meet someone and think, *Oh! There you are. Where have you been?* Intrinsic familiarity times a hundred. I might not yet know who he would be as a *person*, but I knew his spirit. It was one that I had already known wherever we were floating around before we got to these bodies.

Go ahead. Call me hippy dippy.

What they don't tell you is, as magical as it is to feel that baby inhabit a life inside your body, you can *feel the baby move when you're peeing.* Yeah, that's right. On the toilet. Especially if it's a big pee, presumably because the pee was taking up a lot of room and the baby can stretch out after your bladder is empty.

I usually had to lean forward to fully empty my bladder so that I only had to go seventeen times a day as opposed to twenty. That made me feel like I was squishing my baby *up against* my pee, and I feel horrible about that. My baby was better than being squished against pee.

And don't even get me started about the poo. (Too late. You got me started.) There was something about my uterus taking up the majority of my abdominal cavity. Maybe it squished my intestines, so now I could *feel* my poo moving through my tummy. And I'm pretty sure that, if I could feel it, my son could probably feel it. And that's horrible. My baby was stuck being pushed around by poo and pee. If he could get pushed around by that stuff, what would happen when he was out and had to face the kids at school? Would he have a complex about the fact that he couldn't even stand up to poo and pee?

This is the stuff you have time to think about in the bathroom while praying that leafy greens and stool softeners actually do prevent the dreaded hemorrhoids everyone warns you about.

Pregnancy really is a miracle.

Phillip and I opted for as many movies as possible while I was pregnant because we knew the ease of just "going to a movie" would soon end. *Iron Man* was the most exciting movie on the list, but we promised my mother we'd see it with her for Mother's Day (because … Robert Downey, Jr.), so we settled on *Babies*. This film, a documentary about children being raised around the world, completely changed my view of child rearing.

Spoiler alert: I'm going to tell a few stories from the movie, so if you're a freak about being surprised about every little detail, read it anyway 'cause it's super cute.

A baby in Mongolia was born in a hospital, and by "hospital" I mean dirt floor of a hut. A few days later, he was wrapped in a blanket, which was a stiff piece of canvas, and tightly tied up with some loose piece of fabric. The mother boarded the back of a moped and zoomed back to her village. This baby's entire story included video of him almost exclusively alone. Mom was outside farming and caring for the animals much of the day, so he was left to learn and grow alone for hours at a time. He played with chickens, slept with goats, and discovered a roll of paper towels. The point? *He was fine.*

Compared to the baby profiled in a Big City in America (you know the one: Mommy and Me groups, seventy books a day, baby yoga, ridiculous amounts of enunciation), this Mongolian baby actually seemed totally fine! They don't need bouncers, play yards, and swings. This movie proved it for me. Pacifiers? The Mongolian baby used his foot to pacify himself, which turned out to be a very exciting scene in the movie. Toys? The Mongolian baby played with rocks (and occasionally ate them). Diapers? One baby pooped on his mom's leg, and she wiped it off with a corncob.

The Big City baby couldn't say boo without twenty people shouting, "How high?" And when the baby got angry because she didn't want to sing the damn song Big City Mommy was forcing her to learn and hit her in the face, Big City Mom pulled out the "No Hitting" book. The kid was barely a year old.

I realize we have disposable diapers in this country, and we teach our children to read because it's necessary in our culture, but after watching that movie, I felt much less pressure to learn the latest baby sign language techniques. The truth is, barring any interference from spoiling grandparents, my kid would be fine without all the stuff, all the latest and greatest. And if my dogs were to lick my boy directly in his mouth? I'm guessing he'd still make it to college.

This isn't to say I didn't register. I registered the hell out of Target's website. I mean, I'm still American.

And then a funny thing happened. Shortly after watching *Babies* and realizing how very little my baby needed, my sense of peace and well-being vanished, replaced by mind-numbing panic. I was six months pregnant.

Six months, people.

Hadn't I just told our family I was pregnant a few minutes earlier? And wasn't I only ten weeks along when I told them?!

Now I was six months pregnant.

I had three short months to paint his room, figure out what he would sleep in, what kind of diapers he would use, and how many burp cloths I needed to stash in each room of the house. I tried to prioritize. First, I should paint his room.

As I contemplated colors, my mind zeroed in on Charlie barking in the other room. In three months, that would no longer be acceptable. But how would I stop my dogs from barking so much? Should I start warning neighbors, friends, and the UPS man that, if they rang the doorbell, they'd be electrocuted?

A birthing plan. Someone had recently mentioned that. I should get one of those.

I wondered if he was allergic to our houseplants. Those should all be destroyed, I was guessing.

I knew nothing about children's toys, and there weren't many in the house. I needed to get those toys that were vital to his visual development before the three-month mark or he might not ever be able to ... you know ... see. And books! I didn't think I had enough books. Was I supposed to be collecting books like the Big City mom after all? Should I read to him even when he was still trying to remember to breathe in between swallowing gulps of milk?

How was I supposed to organize his clothes? I already organized them—once by level of fancy and once by size-month. Now I was thinking fancy was better, but we should also differentiate between daywear and eveningwear.

Would he ever actually wear shoes that were this small?

I should register for more pacifiers, right?

Did *anyone* know the proper way to use a baby wrap?

The backyard was gated, but the front yard wasn't. This was starting to make me nervous.

He needed more pictures in his room. I didn't want him to feel as if he couldn't have pictures.

Should I try the hypnobirthing class?

I needed to check that child molester website again.

No matter who you are, you give in to some of these Supposed-Tos. I went out and bought all the toys with plastic bags inside of them because "babies like that noise." I registered for and was gifted nearly thirty-five receiving blankets. *Thirty-five!* I had at least eight receiving blankets in every room of the house. I bought or was given three vibrating chairs. Teddy bears, blankets, trinkets, onesies, tiny shoes … all these cute little things. I hate cute little things. I wanted none of it. But I felt as if I was *supposed* to have it all in order to be a prepared mom.

If I could have a real heart-to-heart with Six-Months-Pregnant Erin, I would tell her to let the damn dump of "shoulds" go by. I would tell her to stay conscious and present with that little spirit and know that she would meet his needs. Whether she gave him a natural birth or got a C-section, breastfed or used formula—that stuff didn't matter.

But then again, Six-Months-Pregnant Erin would have probably looked me in the face and ordered another receiving blanket.

Because, let me tell you, it's really damn easy to fall victim to the New Baby Supposed-Tos (even if you watched *Babies*). There comes a point in pregnancy wherein you get big enough that everyone around you fast forwards to the baby being born and home. They then require answers to questions that you suddenly feel pressure to know. People asked me about educational toys, cloth diapers, nipple shields for nursing, postpartum depression, glass bottles, sanitizing bags … I mean, the kid wasn't even going to be able to see more than six inches in front of him, but by all means, let's paint his room.

I got caught up in the Mommies' Underground Railroad. Moms from everywhere gave me piles and piles of their old baby supplies. So not only did I have two brand-new, state-of-the-art vibrating bouncy chairs, I had two older versions of the exact same chair just in case I wanted to have three extra vibrating chairs in the living room. (But you don't have to worry about recalls when it comes to the Mommies' Underground Railroad. If it didn't kill their kids, it won't kill yours.) I was given gobs of clothing, more books than I've read in a lifetime, and boxes of toys. And despite being grateful, I could not for the life of me figure out why these women were just giving me their stuff. Well, let me clue you in on a little secret: this is actually a way for moms to offload all the shit that has accumulated because of their own Supposed-Tos. I'm sure some of it is people feeling giving, but I know when I give stuff away, I'm doing it to get it out of my house.

And in all that time, it never occurred to me that my son might hate swings. (Which he did.) Or that he might hate all brands of pacifier but one. (Which he did.) Or that he might not like any of the baby swaddlers we had. (And he didn't.) I was so caught up in accumulating and arranging things that I felt my baby would need based on what *other people* had told me, that in actuality, I had few of things I truly needed. You know what else? In all that time, in all the advice for how to prepare our physical environment for our children, no one ever considers the work you need to do to prepare your physical *self,* your mental, emotional, and spiritual *self,* for your child. We distract ourselves with eight-dollar glass bottles because, you know, plastic kills!

If you're pregnant and reading this, give yourself a break. Pay attention to what your *body* needs. If you're tired after you eat a meal, then just lie down and stay there until you feel like getting up. Allow yourself to feel what you're feeling, and trust your instincts about what you and your baby need. All the external stuff is cute, some even important, but all your baby needs is you, so be gentle on yourself.

And, for God's sake, don't buy another receiving blanket.

While I received mountains of baby stuff, what I did not receive was pregnancy stuff: maternity clothes.

Up until this point, I'd been getting away with a lot of stretch pants and sundresses. But there comes a point where the bottom of a sundress stretches so far that it almost becomes a shirt, and the stretch pants give in and surrender. My Belly Band still worked, but honestly it got harder and harder to get it on because bending over was pretty uncomfortable. It was time to try actual maternity clothes.

I drove to a popular maternity store to look through the sale section because I don't pay full price for anything. My main objective was shorts. Summer in Florida would not be pretty with an extra Abe inside my belly. The least amount of clothing possible without making one of the local new station's top evening stories was the goal.

I had just found a pair of shorts that I liked and that were on sale when I heard the dreaded, "Are you finding everything okay?" I'm not one of those people who likes help when I shop. I like to shop when I shop, and then I like to stop shopping.

"Yes, I'm all set!" I smiled.

"Okay, well I'm Felisha if I can help you find anything, okay?"

"Sounds great," I smiled again. Felisha walked away. I picked out another pair of sale shorts, and within a millisecond, she was back.

"Can I get a fitting room started for you?"

Admittedly, a fitting room would be helpful. "Sure. That'd be nice," I said. I smiled waiting for her to walk away. Did she? I'll give you three guesses.

"You know, the secret belly-suction-magical-flap (I'm paraphrasing what the thing was called because whatever it was sounded equally ridiculous to what I just wrote) on some of these shorts are really preferred by most pregnant women. I see you chose a shorter ruin-your-life-and-kill-your-baby belly flap (again, paraphrasing) which can sometimes ride up and make you uncomfortable. Would you like me to get you a pair with a secret belly-suction-magical-flap so you can try them on?"

"Sure." *Whatever. Just go away and let me shop.*

The entire time I shopped, Felisha loomed. She watched every choice I made. It had been a while since someone on commission followed me so closely in a store that I wanted to turn around and shout, "Nobody does this anymore, lady. Not even car salesmen!" I took an extra-long time wandering around the store to see if I could lose her and resume my normal shopping pattern. After about twenty minutes, I gave up. "Um, Tracy was it?"

"Felisha! Here, right here! I went ahead and chose a few items similar to the ones you chose and added them to the room."

"Oh, okay. Thanks."

I walked into the dressing room after having chosen three pairs of shorts and two shirts. Guess what was hanging on the rack? *Nine* pairs of shorts, *two* pairs of jeans, and *four* shirts. I stood there, staring at the clothes I hadn't chosen, seething with rage. I couldn't even remember what items I'd chosen anymore.

"Everything fitting okay?" she knocked.

"Yes, yes fine!" I shouted in a frantic tone.

I stood in my regular clothes staring at all the shorts. Finally, I picked up the first pair. I had no idea whether they were a magical flap or a kill-your-baby flap. I tried them on. They didn't fit. I took them off. I did that a few more times, still wondering which ones I had initially chosen.

Then I figured it out.

Price tags.

I had chosen shorts that cost $20.

Felisha had chosen shorts that cost $90!

Ninety freaking dollars. For a pair of shorts that I can wear for six months? I hated Felisha. I hated her shorts, and her jeans, and her tops. I grabbed the pair of shorts I originally chose and headed to the register.

"Oh, you chose these? Well, as long as they were comfortable for you. Can I get you a few more in other colors or—"

"No. No, thank you."

"Are you sure? Because the spring line has—"

"*No.* Felisha, I can't afford more than one pair."

"Oh. Okay." She rang up my shorts. I looked at the little screen and watched a price twice as high as the tag whizzing by.

"Um, Felisha? Is that the right price?" She didn't answer me. She didn't even look at me. She just hurriedly put a bunch of numbers into the computer and the right prices came up. What if I hadn't been looking? Would she have totally over charged me? After pretending that didn't just happen, she asked for my address. "Why do you need my address?"

"So that we can add you to our mailing list."

"I don't want to be on your mailing list. Do you still need my address?"

"No, ma'am. Can I please have your email address?"

"Why do you need my email address?"

"So that we can send you coupons. We send out over four hundred dollars' worth of coupons and discounts to our customers every year!"

"Well, I'm only going to be pregnant until September, so I can't imagine I'll be using maternity store coupons for an entire year."

Felisha finished ringing me up and handed me my bag. I'm pretty sure she was still talking when I walked out. I promptly drove home and ordered an entire maternity wardrobe at Old Navy Online. Not a single virtual employee bothered me.

Bye, Felisha.

CHAPTER 22

Bigger

Weight was still on my mind, which really pissed me off. There's this floating misnomer out in the Universe that, if you're lucky enough to get pregnant, you get to forget about weight. Everyone expects you to be fat, so enjoy it! Right?

Nah. It took one word from my doctor to send me into a complete panic about my weight. But that wasn't all! Other people made comments too! Family members, friends, even strangers commented on my size! It was mind blowing! The nerve!

Okay. Okay. I'll admit it. Once, when I was not pregnant, I made a joke about a pregnant woman's size. And for that, karma seemed to be repaying me *in full*.

A few rules you should know:

- It is never, under any circumstance, funny to call a pregnant girl fatty.
- Don't ask her how many she has in there, either. If there's more than one and she wants you to know that, she'll tell you.
- Don't joke about the new, wider gait she's undoubtedly walking with. If she doesn't walk that way, she'll fall over, and that's just more jokes.
- Even if you like her new booty, legs, or belly, she doesn't want to know that you can tell the difference, so don't comment.

- Stop asking her how she feels. Just take a guess at how twenty pounds suddenly gained all in one spot would make you feel. Then pick something up off the ground for her.
- There is no need to offer her more food. She is pregnant. She has not lost the ability to communicate hunger.
- When you hug her, don't shout things like "Whoa!" or "Look out!" She's aware there is now a person between herself and everyone else with whom she comes into contact.
- Offer her a hand when she tries to get up off a cushy couch. You can also tell her she looks beautiful, amazing, or like she's glowing. Because trust me, the weight is on her mind. She is counting every effing pound. (Excuse my French abbreviation.)

I went for walks every day, I constantly and strenuously cleaned my house to keep up with the ridiculous nesting hormone, I ate small meals every few hours to keep my blood sugar steady, I incorporated plenty of protein and lots of fiber, I drank sixty ounces of water a day, *and I was still* ten pounds further than any baby book ever written says I should be. *Ten pounds!*

On those weight loss shows, don't they have them wear weights while they walk so their bodies think they're heavier so they burn extra calories? I was wearing twenty extra pounds! How was I not burning more calories?!

I know exactly what you're thinking: "Stop it, Erin, I'm sure you looked great." (And if you're not thinking that, shame on you. Have you learned nothing from The Rules?) But the trouble is that it is virtually impossible to be anyone's version of a normal pregnant woman. There is no normal, which is why there are fifty thousand pregnancy books floating around, each describing its own version of normal, and it's why we end up sitting on the couch watching *The Biggest Loser* and sobbing uncontrollably about our abnormalities and eating chocolate ice cream with sprinkles and peanuts and Oreo crumbles while our partners sit helplessly, telling us we're beautiful when we know we look like we should be at the next weigh-in. I wasn't sure if this weight was going to "fall off" because I "chose to breast feed" or because I was "so small before." In the meantime, I needed a lobotomy every time the digital scale added insult to injury by reminding me that not only had I gained twenty pounds, I'd also gained .4 pounds.

CHAPTER 23

Drinking Sugar (For My Health)

Between twenty-four and twenty-eight weeks, pregnant women are asked by their ob-gyns to participate in a glucose screening. You first arrive at the butt-crack of dawn at a neighborhood clinical laboratory. Then, while maneuvering around a number of different levels of sickly people, you approach the sign-in area. Once at sign-in, a nice nurse or phlebotomist hands you a small bottle of juice. Remember the little plastic juice bottles with the foil tops from the diabetes test? That's the one. The one that tastes like someone poured artificial flavoring, water, fifty grams of sugar, and a little bit of feet into the bottle instead of juice. You have five minutes to drink this concoction, and you can't vomit. Then you sit and watch all the people come and go for an hour while your body screams and throws itself into walls, trying to deal with the ridiculous amount of sugar you just ingested. Then the phlebotomist returns to take a bunch of blood while you crash in the chair. Then you drive home (though you might not remember that part). Sounds like fun, right?

My blood sugar had to fall under a certain level in order to "pass" this test. Failing the test by even one point meant I could be diagnosed diabetic or, in my case, a gestational diabetic (pregnant diabetic).

A few days after I endured this ordeal, I received a phone call from a nurse. I won't call her The Worst Nurse Ever. No, I'll abbreviate it and call her "TWNE."

TWNE called me and talked *at* me through the phone to say, "Hi, so we got your labs back and your sugar is *really* high, so you need to go back and take the same glucose test again, only this time you'll have to stay for three hours."

"What does that mean, my sugar is 'really high'? What is the three-hour test? Am I supposed to know what all of this means?"

TWNE didn't really bother answering my questions, but instead said, "Your sugar should be around one twenty but it was one fifty. If you're next test is bad, too, then you'll be diagnosed with gestational diabetes and you'll have to take insulin. I'll send you the form you need to take back to the laboratory. Get that three-hour test done this week. Any questions?"

I mean … yes. I already asked them but you didn't answer them.

"It's pretty common for women in your circumstances—prediabetic diagnosis and PCOS and infertility treatments—to develop gestational diabetes. If it goes untreated, you face side effects—like your baby could grow too big too fast, it could grow an abnormally large head, or could experience fetal demise. Can you give me a fax number where I can send this form?"

Fetal demise.

Say it out loud once so you can hear just how scary it sounds. In the same breath, TWNE told me that my baby could die and asked for my fax number.

When I was growing up, I lost my grandfather, my dad, and an uncle all in two and a half years. My fear of the people around me dying manifested in obsessive phone calls when someone was late, and frantic driving to check on people I loved if I couldn't contact them. When the words *fetal demise* entered my life, they added to the already inordinate fear of my baby son dying inside me or during childbirth. My plan was always to have as natural a birth as I possibly could, but now I just wanted to be assured every day, day in and day out, that my baby wouldn't die.

I set the phone down and stared at the wall, bewildered. My sugar is high? I'm not eating a lot of sugar. Sure, I'm eating more than I was during my fertility diet, but nothing crazy.

The next day, I decided to try a cupcake. I wanted to know what it *felt* like to ingest sugar. And sure enough, within a few moments I felt dizzy. I felt as if my insides were almost hollow, and my brain got a little bit foggy. I didn't quite feel nauseous, but I didn't feel right either.

Two days later, I took my form back to the lab and repeated the process, only this time I had to drink *more* of the drink, stay for *three* hours, and have my blood drawn four times. That's right. I was not metabolizing sugar correctly, so the Western medical world's response was to feed me *more* sugar and then take more of my blood. It sounded crazy to me.

When I completed the three-hour test, I called Old Man Winter. While he wasn't my favorite doctor, I knew he was in charge. I told him what TWNE had said to me. I told him I felt it was completely inappropriate to nonchalantly mention baby death and ongoing medical conditions without any sense of nurture or compassion or concern (especially for me, a new mom with death issues). To my surprise, he apologized on her behalf. He sighed and then told me that perhaps it was time to revisit the conversation of bedside manner with his nurses. He even told me not to worry (a thing he hadn't done before), and that this was all going to be okay no matter the results.

There's that pregnancy confidence again. There's just something about not only advocating for yourself, but also for someone else—someone you're making.

A few days later, TWNE called me with my second glucose test results. She was nicer the second time she called. I'm not sure if she knew I was the one who had ratted her out for being an insensitive mouth breather, but she sure did deliver the news carefully and kindly. "Erin, I've got your results. Are you ready?"

"Um, yes."

"Well, okay, here they are—you have gestational diabetes. And it's going to be okay. We'll help you."

TWNE went on to explain that I had passed the fasting blood sugar test, meaning my blood sugar was fine when I first walked into the lab, but when it came to that unreasonably sugary drink, my body was thrown for a loop. My diet changes would be very minimal since I was already eating a fairly low-sugar diet. She prescribed me one of those at-home sugar-testing glucometers, for free no less! *That should be fun at parties,* I thought. She also made an appointment for me with an endocrinologist.

This endocrinologist was different from the reproductive endocrinologist I had been seeing before (you remember Dr. New York?). I wished I could go back to Dr. New York, but I guess in order to properly treat me, they had to keep things as complicated and uncomfortable as possible.

Of course, I googled so I could figure out what my body was doing now. The placenta—that big sponge in my uterus responsible for feeding Abe everything I ate—apparently had something against insulin. It sent all kinds of hormones picketing throughout my body with signs reading "Stop answering the door *any* time insulin knocks!" I guess cells are really gullible, because they all believed the picketers and locked up tight. It was pretty similar to the prediabetes issues I had while trying to get pregnant, except now my placenta had joined the party. Extra sugar in my body meant extra complications for my baby.

Was I sad? Yeah, pretty sad. And I was fairly scared. My best friend, Darlene, had just given birth to her beautiful, healthy, perfect little boy. I wanted that more than anything in the world. The selfish side of me also just wanted to have a freakin' normal moment. I kept having those pitiful woe-is-me thoughts: "First I can't get pregnant, then I finally do get pregnant and I have to have all kinds of scary extra tests, I gain more weight than I expect, and I have to start watching my calorie intake instead of happily feeding my face the way most pregnant women do. Now I've got gestational diabetes in the third trimester, and the thought of 'fetal demise' is floating around in my head like an angry balloon on a windy day."

Why did the most challenging part of my life have to come precisely at the time when I had virtually no control over my irrational emotions and while the only thing that could really help quell the sadness was a Snickers bar? This was a cruel trick. Cruel.

While all of these emotions swirled around my house like an angry tornado, frustration built on top. Not frustration over "the diabetes" (said in a deep, Southern accent). Frustration over the number of things I could no longer lift, move, and/or carry. And because of this, there was an inordinate number of things on the floor of my house waiting for Phillip to come home every day to pick up. The dog's giant bag of food sat next to the giant dog food Tupperware container on the floor outside the laundry room. One of Abraham's five new swings made it only to the bottom of the stairs in its original box (dragged, like a dead body). The new car seat and stroller lay all willy-nilly on the garage floor waiting for someone to place them somewhere with more dignity. The giant bean bag chair in the living room remained shoved up against Phillip's grandmother's old dresser where the dogs somehow pushed it while trying to reach a tennis ball under the couch. Oh, and the dogs' tennis ball was under the couch. They'd been whining for five days.

It was incredible that turning the "third trimester" corner so quickly resulted in my inability to do half of the things I had been able to do the previous week.

CHAPTER 24

Bonnie and Clyde

After getting the gestational diabetes diagnosis, I had to wait more than a week to meet with the endocrinologist who would decide what the next steps were. This was totally asinine to me. My baby could accidentally grow seven pounds in that time, and I could be like one of those women who had a fifteen-pound baby and no lady parts left to speak of.

In the meantime, my insurance company was nice enough to keep all arguments to itself and send me a glucometer free of charge. The glucometer was really quite adorable. It sort of resembled a stopwatch and came in a little zipper pack that was barely bigger than a deck of playing cards. The little pack butterflied open. On one side was my little glucometer, and next to that was the device to poke my finger. The other side of the pack held all the clean needles and test strips. I decided to name my glucometer Bonnie Bloodchecker—Bonnie for short.

I didn't know how to use Bonnie when I first got her, and because my appointment was days away, I felt that Bonnie and I couldn't yet forge a friendship. But, as it turned out, my sister-in-law Sharon just happened to have an odd affinity (close to an obsessive love) for glucometers. It was a strange and lucky twist of fate that I married into a family that happened to include someone with the ever-elusive Glucometer Fetish. (In fairness, it wasn't really a fetish. She just happened to work for a cardiologist as a medical assistant B.K. [before kids]. She had spent six years helping people learn how to check their blood sugars. Lucky me!)

She showed me how to attach the clean needle to the finger poker, wipe my finger with an alcohol swab, cock the finger poker like a gun, and then *shoot* my finger to get a little blood out.

I could set the needle to different levels so that I could regulate how deep it went, and the first time I did it, I set it way too deep. I yelped as the needle pierced the soft flesh of my finger, but I still managed to turn on the glucometer, stick the test strip in a little runway at the end, and touch my bloody finger to the test strip. The test strip soaked up the blood, and then the glucometer sucked up the test strip to give me a reading. I started checking my blood three times a day.

I had no idea when to check my Bonnie numbers or what they meant, but I figured some would be better than none when I met with this new endocrinologist.

I also started keeping a detailed food journal so that I could see patterns between my blood sugar and what I ate. I wrote down *everything*. In a lined school notebook, I recorded the date at the top of each page and then broke down every morsel I put into my mouth. I started immediately with what I ate for breakfast. An hour after that, I took my blood sugar and jotted the number down in the notebook. Then I ate a snack and then lunch. I wrote down whether I ate half a sandwich or a whole sandwich, two spoons of cottage cheese or a tub.

I thought that if I had all this information with me (the food journal, my Bonnie numbers, detailed questions, meal plans, exercise regimen, etc.) in a neat little folder, the endocrinologist would tell me everything was fine and not to worry. Phillip proudly sat next to me in the exam room at our first appointment reassuring me that my notebook was great. So it came as quite a shock when a tall, curly-haired lab coat walked in, complimented my dedication to health and wellness, and then prescribed me daily insulin injections.

"Great job logging everything so far! We need to keep your numbers under one thirty. We're going to start with a small amount of insulin, and we will increase it throughout your pregnancy."

"Uuuuuuuuuh—"

"You'll give yourself two injections a day, one upon rising and one before bed. My nurse will show you how to administer the insulin for yourself."

"Buuuu—"

"We'll check your levels at a clinic periodically to decide how much insulin to give you in the coming weeks, as your sugars will increase as the pregnancy progresses."

"Flahrg-sah—"

"You'll need to fax in your daily sugars on this little chart every Friday so I can see how things are going. Do you have access to a fax machine?"

"Fax machine."

"Great. And then I'll see you again in four weeks."

I don't even think I'd caught her name yet.

Insulin injections? But I had been checking my blood sugar and writing it all down in my neatest handwriting. How could I be reliant on insulin at twenty-eight weeks? I was the perfect patient and the picture of self-care!

She looked up to shake my hand, and I could tell I was about to cry. Phillip whispered to me, telling me to take a deep breath. I whispered back, "Deep breaths make it worse. Shut up."

She smiled. "We're being preventative. Your baby will be completely fine if we keep our awareness high and stay preemptive with our treatments."

"Abraham," I snapped, as if she was supposed to know my son's name.

"Insulin won't hurt Abraham. He is at no risk for having diabetes after he is born." I, however, would face a fifty percent increased risk of developing Type 2 diabetes later in life, she explained. Great. So my kid would be fine, but his mom would be in a diabetic coma by the time he graduated high school. Not helping.

The endocrinologist shook my hand (I think) and left.

As if choreographed, The Sweetest Nurse Ever (TSNE) popped her head in right after the endocrinologist left and saw my tears. Her eyes were soft and kind, and she held my hands when she told me that I was going to be okay. That only made me cry more, and so she hugged me. I really liked her even though I'd just met her seconds before.

When I finally felt okay enough to listen to her spiel about insulin, TSNE began. She showed me how to unwrap a syringe, stick it in a tiny bottle of insulin, and suck out the right amount. Using her own stomach, she grabbed a little chunk of skin and said, "Like this, and it won't hurt." Her kind eyes and gentle words comforted me even though I couldn't really pay attention.

TSNE put her hand on my shoulder and smiled. She gave me paperwork to fill out every day with my Bonnie numbers and wrote the fax number at the top. The insulin would need to be "upped," she told me, and that this was "normal." I would need to get my Bonnie numbers three times a day and shoot insulin twice a day. That's five shots a day. Five needles. Every day.

And I just felt numb.

In the elevator on the way out, Phillip smiled. "We got this," he said. That helped a little bit. Then he went on. "Come on, babe. You've got too much panache to have a normal pregnancy! We had to shake it up somehow!"

He was kinda right. But it was still too soon.

Someone suggested I name my insulin Clyde, a suitable partner for Bonnie. I liked this. They were both a little evil, but they worked together as such a good team. Inseparable, really.

Next to my bed I set up a pretty glass jar with all my needles and lancets and alcohol swabs. This bedroom—the one where I used to watch *Will and Grace* at eleven p.m. in all my depression, the one where I listened to the train, the one with the bed on which I had lain waiting for Phillip to tell me the home pregnancy confirmed I was pregnant because I was afraid I really wasn't—this bedroom was now feeling like a strange combination of hibernation den and a war zone. I hated that.

Honestly, though, Clyde didn't hurt. He slid right into the side of my belly quietly and quickly. My Bonnie numbers stayed fairly even over the next few days. My fingers, on the other hand … Bonnie mangled my fingers. Four pricks a day, and sometimes I forgot which finger I'd last used. They were sore and peppered with little red dots. I needed a better system. And a manicure.

I tried to keep my blood sugar number under 130, but the truth was I had no real understanding of what my numbers actually meant. A few days into my new normal, I was able to get in to see the nutritionist on staff at the endocrinologist's office. I was supposed to see her sooner, but she was fully booked. I liked that she was booked. In my mind, it meant she was good and worth waiting for.

I packed up my little folder and went to the see the Glinda the Nutritionist (not her real name). She worked closely with my endocrinologist right there in the same building but in a small room. To me it looked as if someone important had given her that room just to be nice.

She was well spoken, smart, and to the point. In simple khaki pants and a collared shirt that looked like something a man would wear to Easter dinner, she looked over my numbers and pointed out where and why they were high. She nodded while I flipped through my notebook to match the dates to the blood sugars and see what I had eaten and when. She was able to help me see the amounts of foods that I should be eating, how often I should be eating, and what to pair with what.

"So if you are going to eat an apple," she said, "the size of the apple should be much smaller than your fist, and you need to eat it with peanut butter or nuts because, even though you need the nutrition of the sugar for your baby, you also need fat and fiber to help slow the absorption of the sugar. You should also be taking your blood sugar levels four times a day, not three." She wrote that down on a pink stickie note and stuck it to my folder.

I would need to poke my finger when I woke up, an hour after breakfast, an hour after lunch, and an hour after dinner, and she gave me a booklet with some dos and don'ts, as well as recipes. I found a few things that I liked eating that wouldn't hurt Abe or me, and I pretty much ate the same thing every day: eggs, bacon, and avocado for breakfast, cheese and turkey for a snack, half a sandwich with cottage cheese for lunch, yogurt and nuts for a snack, and a "sensible dinner" like chicken breast and a vegetable. If I wanted a little treat, I would whip heavy cream with cinnamon and add a few strawberries to it.

With this routine, Abe measured right on par during my next checkup with Annie. He was a very good measurer. Bonnie numbers were fairly stable, and Bonnie and Clyde slowly became a part of the family. I woke up, said good morning to Clyde (sometimes begrudgingly because I'm not a morning person) and a quick hello to Bonnie (I knew I would see her again in an hour), and then went about my day eating only the things that made us happy and healthy and completely miserable because we couldn't have cake.

CHAPTER 25

How You "Should" Prepare

Most days I was very excited for Abe to be here, but there were times when I made a quick run to Target or the dogs barked maniacally at the UPS man and I thought, *Crap. This is going to be really hard with a kid on the outside.* I know, I know: just you wait.

We still spent a lot of time "shoulding" ourselves with three billion receiving blankets and twenty-seven bouncy chairs. We also decided it was important to educate ourselves. We signed ourselves up for a birthing class and a breastfeeding class at the hospital where Abe would be born.

Did you know that a baby turns itself into the right position twice during labor? Yep. Once to fit the head through the pelvis and again to fit the shoulders. The doctors don't even need to tell him to do that. He just does it. (Smartest baby ever already.)

And did you know that if you place a newborn on his mother's chest, eventually he will find her breast and start nursing on his own? If only the La Leche League knew. They'd be scared out of their minds. Job security is tough to come by in this day and age.

If nothing else, these classes were fabulous distractions amidst all the bad news.

It was at the end of our breastfeeding class that we were given a flier for an infant CPR class. This one was free, and we both felt it was important to know just what to do in an emergency situation. But we thought we would learn what to do if the kid choked on a grape. We didn't realize that the class was a veritable bullet-pointed list of everything we should be scared about.

The teacher, a middle-aged pudgy woman who hated her job and had somehow pulled the short straw for CPR class, introduced herself (I'll call her Angry Betty). She proceeded to explain how many children die each year from accidental drownings in bathtubs, parents running over them while reversing out of the garage, and from suffocation due to eating peanut butter straight from the jar. She read dryly from a piece of paper, her perfectly dyed blonde bob never once moving as she terrified everyone in the class for two hours on a Wednesday night.

We learned just how unsafe 90 percent of cribs are and how, if you put *anything* in the crib except for the baby, those cribs jump to 99 percent unsafe.

If you have stairs (which we do) you need two James Bond–proof gates, one at the bottom and one at the top. You need two sets of banisters on both sides, a bottom one for when the child is under three feet tall and a top one for when he has a growth spurt. If you have rungs on your banister, you have to cover them in plywood so the kid can't get stuck in them (a la, the *Growing Pains* episode when Carol Seaver was babysitting and the kid's head got stuck and they used butter and shortening to try to slide him out). So, basically, we would have to rebuild an entire portion of our house.

If there are any flowers, plants, or trees in your yard (and grass—don't forget grass), it needs to be fenced off so the baby can't eat anything potentially poisonous. If you have a baby pool in the summer, you can put one inch of water in it without threatening your baby's life. Never buy a house with an actual pool. If you have one, fence it off and cover it with nets and concrete.

Every piece of furniture you own must be secured to the walls or floors in order to keep it from tipping over and crushing the baby. TVs are especially well known for this and must be nailed, glued, or tied down to an entertainment unit that is, itself, nailed to a wall. (Phillip and I high-fived on this one; our TV was mounted to the wall. Point one.)

Kids should not climb trees, ladders, or tall chairs—or short chairs. They should not eat hot dogs that aren't pureed and must *never* go to sleep wrapped in a blanket. Mobiles are a choking and strangling hazard. Rugs should be secured to floors so children can't trip; actually, just no rugs altogether, because … well … *rugs.*

Babies shouldn't play with keys, writing instruments, or phones as they might stab themselves in the eye, cut their hands, or call someone they don't know. No toy should be smaller than a bread box or something like that. And pets. Get rid of all of your pets. They're all dangerous and could hurt or kill your baby. Charlie and Bella would be in the K-9 court system in no time if we weren't careful.

Now, I may have been highly concerned or even frightened upon leaving this scare fest if Angry Betty hadn't ended on one statistic. She did a slow walk through the group of about twenty-five of us, all seated at tables in a small room with our big bellies. She solemnly but sternly asked, "Do you know the *number one* reason our children die before the age of eighteen in this country?"

We all searched our brains for the top news stories of children dying. Car accidents? Drugs? Abuse? All my education and fancy degrees converged into a peak of a mountain of information in my brain.

Angry Betty stood silently, waiting for one of us to answer incorrectly. Terrified to be wrong and further anger her, we waited. As she announced the answer, she nodded as if to commend herself for sharing this all-too-important and shocking piece of information. "Injuries."

I slowly turned to look at Phillip, who was slowly turning to look at me, so that neither of us could be perceived as overreacting. We made eye contact, immediately began to crack smiles that could have quickly gotten out of control and ended up as laughter. To avoid this, we diverted our eyes to stare directly at the teacher with slight smirks on our faces.

"Seventy percent of the children we lose under eighteen years old, we lose due to injuries. Keep that in mind, people."

Isn't this like saying 90 percent of all divorces are caused by … marital problems?

Or that a majority of all people with a runny nose are suffering from … sinus trouble?

I carried our bag of "scare you" pamphlets into the house later that night and promptly trashed every single one of them, but not without announcing, "Oh! Look at this trash can. Injuries. Injuries written all over this!"

It was all a big joke. I wasn't scared of Abe dying from rugs or Bella. But the truth is that my biggest fear was losing Abe before he even got here. It took such work, such emotional trial, just to get him growing inside of me. I had lost my father, and he was a full-grown adult capable of maneuvering around a swimming pool and a bunch of grapes. I had prayed so hard that this little child would find me, and now he was helpless inside of me. He would have no defenses on his way out, no way to tell me if he couldn't handle the birthing process or if he was having trouble breathing. I could control all the things Angry Betty warned me about, but there was so much else *out* of my control.

And if I thought about it for too long, I lost my heartbeat.

Remember the movie *Babies*? All the important lessons I learned about what Abe didn't and didn't "need"?

I didn't.

Abe's room was coming together nicely. Phillip had chosen a lovely shade of blue from a huge stack of paint samples I'd stolen from Lowe's. (I know these are free, but when you take more than ten, it suddenly feels like stealing.) I taped, and he painted. Then I emptied out an entire upstairs closet in another room for no reason other than the fact that I decided we didn't need anything unless I'd used it in the past five minutes.

I believe, in hindsight, I was entering the nesting phase. I wasn't sure if Phillip ever used anything in that closet, but the urge was too strong to bother asking. And when he was finished painting? Streaky. All four walls were streaky. It looked as though the paint hadn't been mixed thoroughly. So he went back to Lowe's. They gave him a free gallon of paint, and he painted the *entire* room again. Small speed bump on the road to Abe's dwelling being perfect.

Because, you know—he would care.

When the room was painted, we put together his crib and glider (that's a rocking chair for you men out there), and set up much of the baby stuff we'd received so far. We still weren't sure what we were doing as far as decorations, except for an awesome hippo picture Phillip's parents had given us from their own wall. ("Well, he has to have the hippo!") And we still needed to hit up Ikea for a dresser to nail to the wall and floor, and some cute mirrors I could hang close to the floor so that Abe could see how handsome he was.

It wasn't just me who was feeling the effects of Abe's imminent arrival; Phillip got the must-buy-a-baby-friendly-car bug. This isn't an actual bug because, if it was, I may have squashed it without telling him and flushed it down the toilet. However, he did an amazing job of negotiating price and style and even agreed to trade in *his* car so that I could keep my Mini Cooper (which is baby friendly, if you ask me). We bought a 2011 Honda Pilot, which was rugged (so I wouldn't feel like I was in a mom minivan), extremely spacious, and way easier to get the car seat in and out of. (Phillip practiced putting a "baby" in the back seat by strapping in a watermelon. It seemed he was now prepared for child rearing.)

At this point, if our kid moved in the next day, we could handle it. And as my mom says, "Grandma came home from the hospital with your aunt and put her in a drawer. You'll be fine."

The trouble at this stage of pregnancy was that we were unprepared for how difficult it was being completely exhausted at seven months pregnant in the dead of a Florida summer (with gestational diabetes and lower-back pain that felt like a leprechaun was following me around with little daggers in his hands, continuously tripping on his own hooked shoes and shouting, "Oops! Oh, sorry again, m'lady!"). In addition to this, other people didn't understand how I was feeling.

No. I was beginning to think that people enjoyed watching a pregnant woman suffer. Why would I think that? It was the only conclusion I could reach when everyone's favorite thing to say was, "Oh, you just wait …" "Oh, Erin. You have no idea. You just wait!"

Wait for what? Was the next step having my baby feeling little to no excitement over his arrival to this world and being actively resentful of the fact that he kept selfishly waking up to eat? Would all the people who had volunteered to help us by cooking meals and doing our laundry for the first month after Abe's birth suddenly back out because they totally forgot they had to "be somewhere"? Was it guaranteed that, no matter how difficult and frustrating life felt right then in my never-ending search to feel normal, I would still have it worse *after* my baby was born?

Just you wait!

They say it. They all say it. And they cannot be considering just how inappropriate it comes across to the already irrational pregnant woman. Imagine if we applied this logic to other difficult times in life.

The last time you got a paper cut or were in a minor car accident, did your friend look at you and say, "Just you wait! It gets worse"? No. Because you would smack your friend in the mouth or at least apply a devastating wet willy to that insensitive person's ear. Or, if you were diagnosed with a mild case of shingles, would it be everyone's first reaction to say, "Just you wait! Those shingles are only the beginning of your suffering and strife." No. Because you'd rub your shingles all over them and run away laughing and maniacally shouting, "Now you wait, suckah!"

Bottom line is that some women float through pregnancy and others trudge through it the way they'd navigate a pool filled with molasses. I was not a floating pregnant woman. I was a trudger. And at no time did someone insinuating that my future would actually be *worse* than my present help me find the will to do … well, anything.

So, pregnant women, unite. The next time someone says "Just you wait," I want you to look him or her dead in the eye and say, "I know. It's going to be absolute hell when I give birth to the person I grew inside of my stomach and get to hold him in my arms every day. It's going to be terrible to watch him learn, and just unbearable to experience all the ups of downs of parenting with a partner who has chosen to go through it all with me. You're right. It's gonna *suck*!"

CHAPTER 26

Listening to My (Big) Gut

The big fear with gestational diabetes is that babies will be too big, deliver early, and not have sufficient lung development to function. We had to keep a close eye on things, so every two weeks I would go in to see Annie and Old Man Winter.

During one of my visits at around thirty-two weeks, OMW ordered a fetal non-stress test (NST). This test measures the baby's heart rate as well as the mother's contractions. If the baby is moving, the baby's heart rate goes up and down, and the doctor can rest assured that the baby is receiving plenty of oxygen.

I sat in an old brown leather La-Z Boy with my feet up. Annie hooked me up to a printer using several different little "remote controls" on belts around my belly. Each belt sent a message to the printer, which shot out squiggly little lines to let us know Abe's heart rate was normal and I was not in labor. At first, Abraham got annoyed. He kicked like a mule and twisted and turned, almost in an effort to avoid the heart monitor. It took two more nurses to find his heartbeat. We could safely conclude he was stubborn like his mama. Also, he did not appear to be a morning person, again like his mama.

One of the nurses noted that Abe's heart rate was really high, and I snapped, "Well, of course it is! He was sleeping, and you pushed him all around in there!" I put my hand on my stomach between the remote controls and said, "It's okay, bud. You can relax." Within ten seconds, his heart rate went back down to normal. I was obviously some kind of Eastern healer.

Abe and I sat with the remotes for thirty minutes until eventually a nurse came in and said everything looked great according to the scribbles on a long paper print out. I think they made this entire process up, but whatever.

On that same day, OMW wanted to do a quick ultrasound to make sure Abe wasn't too big or sporting the head of an elephant. Of course, it was great to see Abe there on the screen with his big cheeks and long legs. He was such a good-looking fetus.

However, the doctor measured him about twelve times to conclude that he was in the seventy-sixth percentile for weight and height. Translation? He was a giant. And in case you didn't know, I am very much not a giant. I am five feet tall. And right then and there, my childbirth education classes, my Lamaze breathing, the bag of massaging instruments I'd been collecting from friends, my focus objects, my birth plan—all of it blew away like a stack of extremely important papers on a windy, wet day. No point in even running around to try to collect them.

Old Man Winter, almost knowingly, suggested I would need a C-section. He told me that this was typical for moms with gestational diabetes. He went on to explain something about Abe's big head and the way they perform C-sections now, and I didn't hear any of it. I floated out of my body. And I cried. Without tears.

This had not been my plan. This had not been what I wanted. I wanted to deliver my baby. I wanted to scream and to push like I'd watched the women on TV do. I hadn't been able to have any part of getting pregnant or being pregnant in the normal way that I wanted, and now giving birth the way I imagined was being taken away too.

Old Man Winter described how Abe could be too big, and how risky it could be to try to push him out because he might get stuck or stop breathing. He told me how the choice would still be mine, but that he would recommend I not "risk it." The fear that was already brewing inside of me about Abe's survival multiplied exponentially as I began giving up all my hopes and dreams of what having him would look like in favor of just keeping him alive.

I didn't speak while we walked out of the office. I stared straight ahead as I put one foot in front of the other and held my breath.

I called Phillip from the parking lot, but I gave him only the general outline of OMW's suggestion. I didn't want to weigh pros and cons. I just wanted him to know.

I cried all the way home.

After my doctor properly frightened me out of all my birthing options, I tried to spend a good deal of an afternoon lamenting. But lamenting is not *nearly* as fun when you can't eat chocolate or potato chips. So I cut it short and started doing some research.

As the fates would have it, my studies were continually suggesting to me that the road to vaginal birth was not necessarily completely blocked off for me. You see, there may actually be a woman who knew the way straight to Vaginal Birth Lane, a woman who had been living on that very street for quite a while.

This mythical creature's name was Doula. Doula Shmoula. She spent her days advocating for women who wanted to live on Vaginal Birth Lane and who always found C-Section Avenue to be a secondary option, even though it's easier to find. Doula had maps, lists, and a GPS system that she didn't force women to learn to use, but rather used herself to guide them while explaining what these tools meant. It was also her role to explain to Vaginal Birth Lane police and other nasty nay-sayer neighbors that it was not their choice where mothers opted to try to live.

Now, I had never actually met a Doula Shmoula, but I had emailed one several months back. A friend of mine knew her and suggested that I email early in my pregnancy to talk about my birth plan. (You know. Another "should.") Since I had not received an answer from her, I assumed that mythical creatures did not exist, or perhaps just didn't use the internet. I was destined to navigate the confusing streets of Birth Town myself.

What's interesting is that the afternoon I was lamenting, I asked the Universe to send me the answer to how Abe would best enter the world; whatever that method might be, I vowed, I would surrender to it. Low and behold, Doula Shmoula emailed me the very next morning.

Apparently, even mythical creatures have spam folders.

She apologized for having missed my email, and a promising email exchange later, Phillip and I were officially going to meet Ms. Shmoula herself.

As it turned out, she was even more fantastical than the stories would suggest! She was about my age, had long dark hair, and was maternal and nurturing. She worked out of the birthing center (an alternative location to the hospital for giving birth) and was sitting barefoot on an exercise ball when I walked in. Phillip would be meeting us there after work, and I carried both of our low-carb, sugar-free meals, which I had packed.

After a few minutes of small talk, she laid it on me. "I am here as an advocate for you," she said. "I am here to educate you. I am here to help you understand what your options are and to help you change your choices as your labor changes, because it will."

"Okay. Well, I think my plan is mostly to just get this baby out alive and in under twenty-four hours. That's about as far as I've gotten—"

"That's a really good start." She smiled. "Babies come into the world on their own time, and contrary to a lot of doctors' opinions, a vast majority of them can come into the world naturally. But you get to decide how 'natural' you want to be. And I can help you make those decisions while keeping you both safe."

Told you she was dreamy.

Then we started talking about labor and fears. Softly, she said, "You have a lot of fear around losing your baby."

It was a statement, not a question, and that gave me permission to be honest. I let out my breath. "Yeah," I said. "I do."

"Why is that?"

"I have lost so many people in my life," I said, feeling my chest tighten with stupid pregnancy hormonal emotion. I thought of my dad's smile. "I have worked *so hard* to get this far. I don't want to lose him." After a moment, I asked her, "Have you ever lost a baby you were helping to bring into the world?"

"Well, yes," she said simply.

Ooookay, I thought. This woman has *lost babies*. We need to find another doula.

"It does happen, but it's very rare," Doula continued, still in the same calm, soothing voice. "I am not worried about losing Abe. Everything is going to be okay. But I am concerned about your fear. I want you to go into this feeling strong."

Just slightly, I let her serene confidence chip away at my fear. Maybe she was right. Maybe everything *would* be okay.

Phillip joined us shortly after she told me everything would be okay, and as we ate from our perfectly packed Tupperwares, I told Doula about Old Man Winter's assessment and asked what she thought about his strong recommendation for C-Section Avenue. Without hesitation, Doula suggested that we wait until Abraham was ready to come into the world, and that when I went into labor, we would soon know whether he was too big or in the wrong position to come out naturally. And if he was, then guess what? C-Section Avenue it was! Imagine that! We'd wait to see if I *needed* a C-section before we *scheduled* one! Novel idea, no?

This all seemed like a very obvious conclusion, but as I told Doula, when a doctor in a white lab coat tells you there's no other way, one tends to believe. It's not until a gal wearing the sweatpants she wore the night before while delivering a baby tells you that you have options that you snap out of what Phillip called "The Doctor Kowtow."

Was I scared to approach Old Man Winter with *my* plan? Yes. Yes, I was. I was a rule follower. I liked to impress people with how well I could follow rules. I *always* used my blinker and never held the Windex closer than ten inches from the bathroom mirror. And in my weeks of checking my Bonnie numbers and giving myself insulin, I had only forgotten twice. Six pokes, every day, for weeks. Two misses, each by no more than an hour.

There were times I caught myself in the car at the time I needed to check my blood sugar. What did I do? I drove with my knees while I prepped my finger, poked myself, and slid the test strip into the glucometer. Was it rational? No. Safe? Like, not at all. But I was in a trance. I was following any and all rules that would ensure Abe's safe delivery.

But in this particular case, I knew that Old Man Winter's plan was not right for me. And as Doula said, this doctor worked for *me*, not the other way around. (My voice cracked even as I *typed* that sentence.) So I left a message at this office. I kindly explained that it was mine and Abraham's choice how he started his process of entering the world. We wouldn't have control of everything. We knew that. But we wanted to let nature take its course.

To our shock, OMW called back and said he completed understood. No arguments. He just said okay. He wasn't even curt. We were very lucky that he respected our decision, and even more lucky that we had access to a C-section if and when that became a necessary step.

This, my friends, is magic from a woman called Doula Shmoula who would soon rub my back and repeat over and over again, "This is completely normal."

CHAPTER 27

Listening to My (Big) Gut Even Harder

I was still on a very low dose of insulin twice a day. I kept such a close eye on my Bonnie numbers that I could see the patterns and rhythms of my blood sugar clearly. After about two every afternoon, my body suddenly started processing sugar more efficiently. How did I know this? Because my blood sugar shot up the moment I had a piece of toast with peanut butter in the morning but remained a beautiful 115 every night after dinner, even if dinner contained carbs and sugar. For some women it's oranges that cause their blood sugar to skyrocket. For others, its tomatoes. For me, it was all about the timing.

Since the amount of insulin I was taking was hardly enough to make a dent, and because my blood sugars weren't rising, as the endocrinologist had suggested they would as pregnancy went on, I knew most of my success was coming from the way I was eating. Glinda the Nutritionist's suggestions were keeping me healthy.

Every human body is different. At this point I was so keyed into mine, I knew exactly when and why my blood sugar would spike. I faxed my weekly Bonnie numbers to the endocrinologist who said I didn't need to increase my insulin because my numbers were so good. Not everyone's body responds this well to a change in diet alone with diabetes. I was incredibly lucky that my routine was working.

So I wondered why I needed to continue taking Clyde with Bonnie at all? Did I really *need* insulin, or was it a medication I was pumping into my body because this was the protocol for a woman like me? I really didn't want to take more medication than I had to, but I also wanted to keep Abe safe.

But Clyde was one of those guys who assured me the poke marks would all be worth it if I just kept up our relationship; after all, he liked to remind me he was only one that could help me with gestational diabetes. There were many a night when I looked him in the eye and said, "I can't do this, Clyde. I don't feel right about it." And he just slyly responded, "It's your choice, but do you really want to hurt your baby? I need you, and you need me, and we both know it." How was I supposed to argue with that?

Well, I'll tell you how. One morning, I decided to do an experiment. I woke up, got my number from Bonnie, and walked right past Clyde. I didn't even wake him up to tell him I was leaving. I didn't want the arguing or the guilt he'd try to poke me with. I just left.

I didn't want to just stop taking insulin without consulting a doctor, but within twenty-four hours, I could see that my blood sugar remained on point even without Clyde. The next day at my OMW appointment, my measurement was perfect and my NST was easy as pie. Sugar-free pie.

I decided I needed to call the endocrinologist and let her know that I would keep myself healthy with diet alone and only take the insulin again if I couldn't control my blood sugar unless there was a huge risk factor I was missing.

(Warning, alert, and caveat: If you have been diagnosed with gestational diabetes and prescribed insulin, *do not stop taking the insulin.* While I felt that the insulin wasn't necessary for me to keep myself and my baby healthy, it is necessary for *many, many women.* Modern medicine is a gift. Be grateful for it and use it as you need it.)

And then the poo hit the fan.

Before I could call her, TSNE (The Sweetest Nurse Ever, in case you've forgotten) called to let me know it was time for a hemoglobin A1c blood test. This is a quick and simple test that looks at red blood cells and calculates the average sugar percentage in your body for the past three months. Anything between 4.9 and 6.0 is normal. Mine had been 5.1 several months earlier; totally normal. But she wanted me to take another to get an update. Rule-follower that I am, I didn't ask questions. I took my veins down to the local bloodsuckers that day, who actually knew me *and* Abe by first name, and left a little sample.

Later than *same day*, TSNE called back and left me a message. "Hi, Erin. Dr. Endo said your hemoglobin A1c went up, and she wants you to up your dosage of insulin starting this week. Call me back. Thanks. Bye."

Several things wrong with this message:

1. Would I ever talk to the actual endocrinologist again or just to TSNE?
2. TSNE never mentioned what my A1c percentage was now. I'd be completely panicking about that until I got back in touch with her.
3. I hadn't taken insulin in two days now. My blood sugar looked fine, but I was terrified to admit my decision to stop taking the insulin to the nurse!

I called TSNE back, and she told me my A1c was 5.6, and then she immediately had to run and "would call me back to answer more questions." Now, I'm not sure how good you are with numbers, but to me, 5.6 still appears to fall within the "normal range." I mean, double-check my math, but ...

I didn't know any friends who would understand why I was so angry. Then a little song began to play in my head. "When a doctor's nuts, and you need some guts, who ya gonna call? Doula Shmoula! When they don't make sense, you need good defense. Who ya gonna call? Doula Shmoula!"

I called Doula and rattled off the whole story.

"Okay," she said calmly. "I agree. It doesn't quite make sense yet. Let's get more information from your doctor so we can see where she's coming from."

She helped me formulate my questions (Why are you recommending insulin? Is 5.1 to 5.6 a big jump? Is there lab variability? Do my consistent Bonnie numbers mean anything?). And she armed me with a little pep talk about trusting my instincts while being open to the professional opinion of my doctors. And when TSNE called back, I was ready. An informed patient, I offered up my questions and assured her that I was glad to take the insulin as long as I understood why.

First, she was appalled that I wasn't taking insulin, and second, she couldn't answer any of my questions except to say that she'd had no idea I wasn't on insulin. Finally, she released the biggest, most frustrated sigh

I'd heard since I last learned we were out of cottage cheese and said, "Well, I guess I'll have to pull your chart and discuss your questions with the doctor, because I don't know the answers."

Um … thank you? For doing your job? TSNE wasn't as sweet when I wasn't crying in the exam room.

It was nearly three in the afternoon on day two of no insulin when the phone rang again. "Sure, yes, I'll see if she's available," I heard Phillip say. "Erin? It's the sweetest nurse ever."

Darn. Darn. Double darn.

I had that half-adrenaline, half heart palpitations thing going, hoping that I could stay calm enough to remember all of my questions and make sense in my reasoning.

"Hi, Erin. How ya doin', babe?" she asked.

Wait. Babe? Hmm. This was new.

"I'm doing just fine, thanks. How are you?"

She skipped the answer and told me she'd pulled my file and spoken to the doctor. She went on to say that Dr. Endo had no idea I wasn't on insulin. (Well, surprise, surprise. Dr. Endo hadn't spoken to me in six weeks. But who wants to dredge up the past?) And then she said, "And Dr. Endo said that's fine."

Wait. Come again? Dr. Endo didn't argue?

"Dr. Endo said, as long as you're keeping your daily numbers in check, there's no need to be on insulin now."

This sudden compliance with the validity of my concerns *completely* blindsided me. My first instinct was to say, "Now you listen to me, Sweetest Nurse Ever …" but I didn't need to.

"So, anyway, Dr. Endo said that if your numbers do start to go up, we'll need to revisit the insulin, but for the meantime, you're doing a great job with the diet and you don't need to go back on it."

"Oh," I said. "Okay, great. So there's no concern about my sugars?"

"Nope."

"And she knows my A1c went up?"

"Yep! But it's still within normal range, and it tends to go up a bit during pregnancy anyway. You're all set. Just keep faxing in those numbers every week and let us know how you're doing, okay, dear?"

Dear? Who are you?

I hung up the phone and sat in stunned silence for a moment. Phillip was waiting for me to tell him everything. When I gave him the other side of the conversation, he smiled and raised his hand in the air. "High five! Team Abe! Way to be an informed patient who thinks for herself and listens to her instincts!"

Ha! Yeah! Booyah! Abe and I were fine! I felt so intensely proud.

Now, none of this is to say that I wouldn't have lunch with Clyde again if my baby's health depended on it. We are lucky enough to live in a country with immediate access to life-saving medical solutions, after all. But somewhere along the line, we can easily forget to think for ourselves instead of nodding and carrying our prescription forms to the pharmacy.

So Abe and I would continue to live a protein-rich, insulin-free life together. Until, of course, he chose to start living it separately from me. Then I would eat pie.

All. Day. Long.

CHAPTER 28

Labor Is Easy

I was now going to Old Man Winter's office twice a week for the NST. Every nurse knew me, and I had the routine down pat: walk in through the small lobby, walk past the exams rooms and down the hall to the NST room, get into the uncomfortable recliner, hang out as they covered me in cords and agitated Abe until his heart rate went up enough times in twenty minutes to consider him "reactive." Reactive meant that the lines on the paper printout from the machine looked like mountains. Abe hated this. I hated this. It was uncomfortable and took at least an hour. I knew he was active. He jumped around in my belly all day, and my ribs could prove it.

On one particular day, I sat there all wrapped up in cords, waiting for Abe to make enough mountains on the paper printout to prove that he was still fine. When the nurse walked in, she was very pleased at all the mountains Abe had made on her printout. But more than that, she was surprised by another mountain range.

"Is he kicking you a lot?" she asked.

"Well, yeah. I mean, he's definitely moving around in there. Why?" I asked.

She sat and watched the printout for a minute or so. Finally, she said, "It looks like you're having contractions. Are you feeling them?"

"Me?" I asked. Admittedly, this was a dumb question.

"It looks right here like you had a contraction." She pointed to a mountain. "You're not feeling them?"

"No, I'm not feeling them." *Kind of awesome if I am having contractions,* I thought. *Labor is* easy.

She asked me to move to Room 2, and I met her on the exam table. She measured my belly. Thirty-five weeks, dead on. She pushed around and asked about pain, then sat down and opened my chart. Then came the words any perfectionist kills to hear.

"You know, Erin," she said, looking up from my chart, "no other patient in the last fifteen years I've worked here has ever kept her sugars so consistently logged and level as you have."

Some women like it when men compliment their bodies. Others love to hear that they're kind, selfless people. I swoon over being commended on my rule-following ability.

"It's probably a good idea for us to check you and make sure you're not dilated," she added.

I lay back, pulled off my underwear, threw my feet in the stirrups, and probably said, "Giddy up." Modesty was no longer my strong suit.

She walked in and slapped on some plastic gloves and gently felt around while I waited for her to tell me nothing was going on and she'd see me on Tuesday for my next NST.

"Oh," she said.

This is where I tell you that, if you are a medical health professional of any kind, you never ever say "Oh" to your perfectionist, over-thinking, rule-following patient.

"What?" I asked, half sitting up and looking down, as if I'd be able to see something.

"I'm not going to check all the way so I don't encourage dilation, but I think you're already about a centimeter. And you're definitely thinning."

Short translation? Labor had begun!

Long translation? The baby sits in the uterus. The cervix is the long, smooshy opening at the bottom of the uterus. It stays tightly closed throughout pregnancy, but when it's time for the baby to come out, it plays a little game of peek-a-boo and opens up a tiny bit at a time. The smooshy part also gets a little bit thinner as the baby naturally moves down and pushes on the tube.

Now, labor can begin weeks before you actually pop the kid out, but still. My body, with a million doctors telling it that it might never handle this on its own, had started doing *exactly* what it was meant to do. I almost cried on the table. I was so unbelievably happy. (I had also cried earlier that day when I realized that Phillip had bought me two tubs of cottage cheese, not just one. Nonetheless, it was a poignant moment.)

I was only thirty-five weeks, so the doctors weren't quite ready for me to give in and just let Abe fly out. I was ordered to modified bed rest. Basically, I needed to lie down whenever possible, but if I had to make a sandwich or go to the store, I still could. They should rename modified bed rest "Dream Come True."

I spent the weekend relaxing on the couch, watching Dr. Phil reruns, and recording my food and blood sugar numbers. Doula Shmoula called on Saturday to see how I was feeling, and when I told her I was on the Dream Come True plan, she approved. "Just lie low," she said. "You're nearing the end. Enjoy this part."

And, oh, did I enjoy doing nothing. By the time you reach maximum baby capacity in your belly, nothing feels better than rolling onto your side and taking the pressure off your back. I probably let out more *ooooohs* and *ahhhs* that weekend than I had on my honeymoon.

On Monday night, I made a simple dinner of chicken and broccoli with a salad and served it to Phillip when he got home. We sat together at the dinner table casually chatting when, without warning, my back muscles began to tighten. Those muscles that wrap around your lower back and attach to your sides felt like they were constricting my kidneys and making it hard to breathe. It was an incredibly slow-moving and odd sensation. Phillip was chatting with me about his day, and I interrupted him to say, "My back hurts, suddenly."

"Oh," he replied. "You want me to rub it?"

"No," I said. "I'm fine."

Phillip kept talking while the tightness in my back slowly spread around to my sides. My attention sort of drifted away from the table, and I stared at the wall. His voice started sounding like a quiet Charlie Brown's mom. Then the front of my belly started cramping, and within in a few seconds, it felt like a huge belt was being tied around my midsection. While Phillip talked, I froze like a statue with my hand on my fork. I got a little bit hot and a little bit dizzy. Finally, Phillip stopped eating and talking long enough to notice I'd become a wifesicle.

"E? You all right?"

"Yeah," I said. I wasn't eat-your-dinner-I'm-normal all right, but I was all right. I took a deep breath, against the will of my diaphragm, and finally the belt started to loosen. I picked up my fork and ate dinner like nothing had happened. It was a little out-of-body.

Nearly the same thing happened at lunch the next day.

When I went in to Old Man Winter's later that day to get a mountain range update, I stopped him in the hallway to ask about that feeling I'd had. Twice.

"Oh, yeah?" he asked with a little smile. "Sounds good. Those are real contractions."

"Really?" I asked, a little louder than necessary.

"Sounds like it. Make sure you time them if you start feeling them often."

"I had real contractions? Like to have a baby?"

"Yep. It's normal."

Ha! Imagine that! Normal! I had done something else that's normal!

"Wow!" I exclaimed. "I'm a centimeter dilated and I had real contractions!"

Old Man Winter smiled and moved on to his next patient because I was making him uncomfortable. He saw this happen every day, so if I was having contractions and dilating a centimeter, he wasn't that impressed. I was smiling as if someone had bought me a huge ice cream and I was actually allowed to eat it.

"Any other questions or changes?" the nurse at the front desk asked me.

"Oh yeah, one more." Now this one I was a little confused about, and now that I was back in the lobby, I was conscious of the fact that other people were around to hear me ask. "There's been a lot of ... stuff ... coming out of ... my lower regions."

"Okay. What color?" she asked.

I looked around to see if anyone was listening. As if anyone in the gynecologist's office would be shocked and appalled that I was asking a question about my vagina.

"Yellow," I whispered.

"Oh, that's your mucus plug. You're slowly losing it. Also normal."

"My mucus plug? I'm a centimeter dilated, I've had real contractions, and my mucus plug is falling out? *Should I be admitted?*"

Modesty gone.

"It's all normal," she said with a laugh. "You're fine. It could be weeks. Just go home and relax."

I couldn't understand how everyone was so casual with all this information. This meant we were on our way to having a baby, people! This was it! Shouldn't there be some kind of confetti or a presentation of beautiful flowers or *something*? A banner releasing from the ceiling that read "You're in labor!" and a guy in a plaid suit with a microphone announcing my name and leading me off to get my lifetime supply of receiving blankets (which I already owned)? If I ever become an ob-gyn, I'm going to have streamers and noisemakers all set up in a special room where women find out they're in the early stages of labor. We deserve this.

Chapter 29

The Home Stretch

In the ongoing quest to make my life difficult, I found out as I was leaving the office after my NST that Annie and the endocrinologist had engaged in a letter-writing war over whether or not I should have to visit a high-risk doctor again during my final weeks of pregnancy. The endocrinologist insisted it was necessary (because she knew me *so* well and had spoken to me so many more times than *once*), and Annie saw no reason for it as she had treated me for nine months. But on a Wednesday afternoon, I got a phone call requesting that I get my last ultrasound with the high-risk doctor. I considered putting up a fight about this but decided it just wasn't worth arguing at this point. I begrudgingly agreed.

Phillip and I drove to the hospital where we'd initially met with Tall Doctor back when we first found out we were pregnant. Phillip drove us through a lot very confusing parking garages, and I waddled my way through an endless chain of hallways and elevators to get to the office. It hadn't seemed this long the first time we were here. It made me wonder why the architects of this building hadn't positioned any and all OB offices near the entrance so we preggos would be spared the exhaustion of a half marathon to visit a doctor we didn't really want to see anyway.

We finally arrived. I was immediately led to an exam room by a nurse who had clearly never been pregnant based on the rate at which she was walking. She was tall with long dark hair, but I can't tell you what her face looked like because I'm not sure she ever looked at me. Phillip stayed behind me, and I caught up to her about thirty seconds after she made it to the door of my exam room. Inside, I plopped down in the nearest chair to catch my breath. Phillip stood in the corner.

"I'm Dr. Stone's nurse," she said. "I'm going to ask you some questions about your medical history."

You can imagine my uncontrollable jubilance at having to give another medical professional my medical history. I answered all her questions, wondering why there wasn't some database somewhere that contained all my medical history for all these information-hungry people. You can get my address and favorite food off the internet in three clicks. Why not what drugs I'm allergic to?

As with all medical professionals, to this nurse I resembled a giant checked box with "Gestational Diabetes" written next to it. She described my risks, including a stillborn baby (thanks for bringing that up again), and reiterated how incredibly important it was that I keep my sugars under control. As she spoke, Phillip could feel me prickling. I wanted to stand up and yell, "*Lady! I kicked insulin's ass. My blood pressure is better than most Olympic athletes' blood pressure. I haven't had ice cream in six months. There's your medical history.*" While I didn't say any of that, my face apparently did, so she sped up the questioning. This was, admittedly, not my shining moment.

I was asked to lie down on the exam table, pull my shirt up, and wait. After a few college flashbacks, I followed directions and waited another fifteen minutes for someone else to show up. The new woman—we'll call her Fast Frieda—walked in and began measuring my stomach and covering my belly in ultrasound jelly before she even mentioned her name. Actually, she never did say her name. I had to ask.

"What's your name?"

"Fast Frieda," she said.

"Oh. I'm Erin."

We made a real connection.

Within about thirty seconds, she had the ultrasound machine booted up and was scanning my belly with her wand. "Femur, looks good. Heart, looks good. Head's down. Here's a foot. There's his package." (She really said that.) "Head is big. Okay, all set. The doctor will be in in a moment."

By this point I was thinking, *Hello? I came to you people because you're specialists. You're* special! *Do something* special!

That was when Dr. Stone walked in. Dr. Stone was apparently Javier Bardem's incredibly hot twin brother with an unbelievable Spanish accent. I was so happy to see Dr. Stone. He shook my hand and introduced himself, even asked me my name and looked me in the eye and asked how I was doing. He completely redeemed his staff with his smoky gaze alone.

Dr. Stone began looking through the pictures on the screen with me, and I listened to his pronunciation of every word, big and small, and probably giggled more than I had since high school. Phillip thought this was pretty much one of the coolest doctors ever too. Dr. Stone answered his iPhone in the middle of our conversation, hung up, and said, "That was my wife. If I don't answer, she gets pissed off. You understand," he added, motioning to Phillip. We loved this guy.

And I loved him even more when he told me what he saw: a six-pound, eleven-ounce baby boy in the fifty-third percentile, measuring exactly where he should. His head was the only big part of him, but it was in the right spot and facing the right direction. He performed a brief physical exam and told me I was almost three centimeters dilated (my cervix smooshy-tube was open almost three centimeters). He told me my sugars were fine, the placenta was fine, and the baby was fine, and not to worry. And then he looked at me and said, "You know what you need to do? Stop checking your sugar so much. Your sugars are fine. Relax."

How much did we love him?

He checked our due date using an app on his iPhone and shook both of our hands before congratulating us and leaving the room.

This was the home stretch.

The last days of pregnancy were very strange. My intense need for this to be over was almost completely overpowering. I couldn't focus on much besides nesting and preparing myself. I had worked from home through my whole pregnancy, albeit part time, and I could work up until the day I delivered. It wasn't as if I had to go into the office or even get dressed. Or sit up. But, suddenly, it became incredibly taxing to think about work. The smallest, most mundane task that didn't include preparing for Abraham was like asking me to run a marathon in my bare feet. (People do that.)

They say that, in the wild, mother animals go into a cave or a far-off place when they're ready to deliver. In fact, even animals at the zoo halt their own labor until they get away from the crowds of people so they can hide in a safe place. I suppose my mind was telling my body it was time to find a cave. There was no arguing with this force. There was no amount of perfectionism that could convince my body to do anything but hibernate and wait. I had a really nice cave with some unbelievably soft sheets and air conditioning. And one day, I finally turned on my work email's automatic responder and let all the clients know that it was time for me to retreat.

I was almost three centimeters. I was thirty-seven weeks pregnant. And there were other encouraging numbers measuring our progress as well. I surrendered to the fact that this last phase of pregnancy could last three weeks or more, and there was not a darn thing I could do about it.

On a Thursday afternoon, I went in for my NST (aka worthless time spent sitting in the uncomfortable chair waiting for Abe to move). While I was hooked up to the machine, I started having contractions. They didn't hurt at all and made lovely mountains on my side of the paper printout. Immediately after the NST, I had an ultrasound to check Abe's amniotic fluid and growth.

"You haven't delivered yet?" asked a nurse as I walked by. Isn't that an adorable thing to ask a woman who is thirty-seven weeks pregnant?

Suddenly, Old Man Winter waltzed in, completed an ultrasound in six seconds, and announced that I was four centimeters, in active labor, and must be admitted to the hospital immediately.

Um, what? I'm not contracting regularly. I don't even feel most of them. Don't I have to have contractions to be in labor?

"Um," I said eloquently, "I'd really rather go home."

Old Man Winter shook his head. He planted his feet. He faced me as if he were going to strap me to a chair and force me to be admitted. Annie walked in behind him and she seemed much less concerned.

"She lives two miles away." Annie chuckled toward OMW, glancing down at my chart before offering me a smile. "She'll be fine."

Old Man Winter glowered. "Well, I don't want her to drive home with contractions."

"She can't feel them. Can you feel them? She can't feel them."

"If her water breaks, she could go fast."

"She's not going to deliver at home. She can come back in the morning and go on the NST again if she doesn't deliver tonight."

All the while, I lay on the exam table wondering if I was still in the room. Eventually, the two decided it was safe to send me on my way. I praised God and called my mom.

"Hey, Mom. I think it's time."

"Oh my god, bah fudge forty heat bingle fine chock," she replied.

She was really excited.

Somewhere in there she told me she was going to pack a bag and drive the three hours to our house.

I also called Phillip, who was excited but, like me, felt like I'd been dilating and having contractions for so long that this was just a red-alert that would result in more waiting.

I felt fine and fairly normal as that night came and went. I drove back to the doctor's office the next morning. My mom offered to come, but since I'd had no contractions for the previous eight hours, I felt confident I would be sent back home (which was what I desperately wanted). In the back of my mind, I kind of hoped to stay home long enough that I just accidentally gave birth to Abe there. After all, I had Doula Shmoula. While she wouldn't do any of the medical stuff, she would know what was happening to me in the moments I'd have absolutely no idea what my body was doing. She would know how to get me in the positions that would help Abe move most comfortably out of me and into the world. If they admitted me to the hospital, I wouldn't get to labor in my tub or on my birthing ball or on my bed or anywhere that was comfortable and serene to me.

Annie hooked me up to the NST machine that Friday morning, and I began to read my book when suddenly ... a contraction.

Seriously?

I hadn't had any contractions in eight hours, and I was getting one in that chair!? Well, certainly one contraction wouldn't be enough to send me to Labor and Delivery.

A second contraction five minutes later. Now? My contractions couldn't wait until lunch?

A third, five minutes later. *This is just great,* I thought. *I'm contracting regularly but* only *when I sit in this uncomfortable chair.* Annie came back in and looked at my mountains.

"Oh! Wow!"

"I know, but I swear, I haven't had a contraction since yesterday. It's only in this chair that I have contractions."

"Mmm hmm," she said not paying attention to me, reading the mountains as if they were hieroglyphics.

"Honestly. I'm not in labor. These are the only contractions I've had. It's this chair. *It's this chair!*" I gave the arm a light slap for emphasis. "If I want to have the baby, I'll just come right back and sit here, I swear."

She smirked, half believing me and half assuming I just wanted to go home. "If you are any more dilated, I'm going to have a hard time justifying sending you home. Let's check you out."

That seemed like a good compromise. She checked me. Four centimeters. Same as the day before. I breathed a deep sigh of relief. I was going home again.

CHAPTER 30

The Feeling of Failing

After another day of no contractions, I started to get frustrated. Come on! Four centimeters? People get epidurals by four centimeters! I called Doula Shmoula to complain.

"I don't know what to do!" I whined. "I feel like I'm in labor, but maybe I'm not. I just have no idea what is happening!"

Calmly, she asked, "What do you want to eat?"

I stopped my pacing. For a second, I wasn't sure she was talking to me. "What?" I asked. "I don't have any idea. Why are you asking me that?"

"Why don't you cook something you really want to eat?" she suggested, nonplussed. "Don't worry about sugar, don't worry about anything. Just go cook something fun. Something *you* want."

This made no sense and also seemed like a really good idea. So I snapped out of my funk, watched the Food Network, and finally decided on a chicken and pasta dish, followed with homemade crepes. I covered them in whipped cream and strawberries and didn't check my sugar.

My mom was in the living room. I was standing in the kitchen with Phillip, eating crepes right there at the counter. They melted in my mouth, and I closed my eyes in bliss. I felt free. Without realizing it, I was nurturing myself and my own body in the way that it needed to be nurtured at that time—not the way the books said or my blood sugar said or my doctors said. Just in the way that felt good. And when I was able to just do something for me, I wasn't panicked anymore. I just felt good. And feeling good felt really good.

I slept well and woke up disappointed the next morning. By this point, I was beginning to resemble a fat Eeyore: "Woe is me. I guess I'll just be pregnant forever. Nobody seems to care anyway."

My friend sent me a link to Deepak Chopra's Twenty-One-Day Meditation Challenge. I didn't have anything else to do, so decided I would try to meditate on labor. (I can be hippy dippy.) I sat, holed up in my room, sitting in the lotus position on my bed, as Deepak told me to watch my thoughts float. It was super hard to concentrate:

"Right here, there is only right now ..."

Mmm, do I smell pancakes? Is Mom making pancakes? No. Wait. Clear my mind. Was that a contraction? Clear my mind. Contraction! *Wait, did I make that up? Did I just feel one? No, I didn't. That was pancakes. Right. Clear my mind. Float back to the now. Here and now. There is only now. I wonder if that was a contraction earlier, though. I should probably open my eyes and look at the clock to see if I can time them. But then I'll break my concentration on "the now." I'll just peek with one eye. Then it's right back to the now. Seven forty-four in the morning. Okay, remember that. Back to the now. I wonder how long this meditation is? I should have looked at the time before I started. Then I'd know how long I had to sit here in "the now." Is that a contraction? Or a cramp ...* Contraction! *Right? Is it?*

This went on for thirty minutes until I finally got up and took a shower. As I enjoyed the hot water splashing on my thoroughly pregnant body, I decided I would get out and invite all of our friends over for lunch. I felt as if I could easily be fooled, clearing my entire schedule in anticipation of Abe's arrival. No way, labor. You won't fool me.

Contraction!

At least, I was pretty sure it was a contraction. I was putting on my clothes, and I just continued on, drying my hair and getting ready for my day. I was not falling for this. I was going to the grocery store to pick up some things, and then I was making lunch. But then ...

Contraction!

They didn't even hurt. They felt like big hugs. On my way toward the front door, I casually mentioned to Phillip that I was feeling contractions, and he stopped me. "We have to call Doula Shmoula!" he exclaimed.

"No, no, don't be so gullible," I said, grabbing my bag. "This is a trick. It's not labor. I'm going to the store."

"Well, I'm coming with you! Your water might break."

"Fine."

Contraction!

Phillip immediately pulled up the contraction timer app on his phone, which he'd downloaded weeks before. He started timing. As soon as each one was over, he announced how far apart they were, as well as duration.

"Six minutes, lasted forty-five seconds!" he said while we were in the spices aisle. "Good one!"

When the woman at the checkout counter asked me when I was due, I smiled and said, "Now. I'm in labor now." I mainly did this for the shock factor, not because I thought I was actually in labor. It worked. Her jaw dropped, and that made me happy. I'd been waiting to say that for nine months.

Contraction!

When we got back home, Phillip asked me if I wanted him to cancel lunch. I explained that, if he cancelled lunch, we would sit around waiting for contractions and they'd stop. So all of our friends piled in with subs and smoothies. My mom traveled back and forth from the living room to the kitchen with napkins and cups. I had a small bowl of fruit from the store, a strawberry-and-banana smoothie, and a tall glass of ice water. We watched *The Hangover* and tossed jokes back and forth.

"Zack Galifinakis and Erin have the same size stomach!" Howard said.

"Oh! This is the scene with Mike Tyson! Erin, don't watch. You'll laugh and break your water."

I was still contracting regularly, but I was easily breathing through them and getting back to the movie.

But Phillip couldn't take it anymore. He sat up like a Jack Russell waiting for me to drop food every time I breathed. He called Doula Shmoula, who agreed it was time for her to stop by the house and hang out for a bit. *Fine, waste her time*, I thought. *But I'm not in labor.*

About an hour later, Doula Shmoula arrived and gave me a big hug. "See?" she exclaimed. "I told you eventually you'd go into labor!"

I'd been contracting since about eight that morning. It was now two in the afternoon, and Doula held the space. She gave us the sense that a professional was in the room and we could all relax. While my friends watched YouTube videos and played games on their phones after *The Hangover* ended, Doula sat and smiled at me. She noticed each time I felt something different happening, almost before I did. Without saying anything or making a fuss, she let me know with her face that I was fine and not to worry.

It was uncanny how brilliantly she anticipated my needs, handing me water before I asked and cutting some of my fruit into smaller bites because I was silently infuriated that anyone would think another human could fit a piece of pineapple that large in their mouth.

It felt like a totally normal day, except that every five minutes I stopped participating in order to breathe.

At about four o'clock, contractions got a bit stronger. My back wasn't involved as much anymore, but the tightness in my belly was way more noticeable. The contractions didn't exactly hurt, but they were strong enough that I absolutely had to stop and breathe through them. At this point, they almost felt like giant foot cramps without the intense pain. Doula suggested I lean on my birthing ball (basically a large, inflatable exercise ball I'd bought with a gift card from TJ Maxx). My friends, good instincts and all, decided it was time to pack up and go.

"Welp, I'm gonna head out," one said. "Yeah. I've gotta run to make a call about a property," another said. We gave hugs and smiles, still almost pretending that I wasn't in labor and my whole life wasn't about to change. Phillip turned off the TV and put on some of my favorite music: a little hip-hop compilation, then some Sister Hazel. He fed me melon and water in between contractions. At this point, it felt as if the belt around my waist was pulling really tight and then loosening every few minutes.

Doula Shmoula was key. She had all kinds of creative positions for me to try. I leaned forward on the birthing ball, I stood up with one foot on a stool, I leaned forward against the back of a chair. At one point, she told me to go sit on the toilet in a squatting position. Some of these positions gave me great relief, and some of them increased the pressure so much that my teeth chattered uncontrollably. I started to feel more than pressure. I started to feel a little bit of pain. Phillip held my hands as I walked from room to room, and he stared at me like a deer in the headlights.

"She's fine," Doula would say. "Focus on her movements and go with her flow."

"Shouldn't we go to the hospital?" my mom finally piped up. I could tell she was getting nervous too. "I mean, when do we go?"

"Erin will know when to go." Doula smiled reassuringly.

It was not reassuring to anyone in the room. Not even me. I didn't know when to go!

Doula was trying to help me position Abe's head to continue the forward progression of labor and make it as easy as possible for him to make his debut, but I didn't care about the mechanics. I just enjoyed that someone understood what was happening to me and was guiding me through the process. I couldn't think past the breathing.

It had now been about twelve hours since my contractions started, and things felt intense. Doula suggested it was time to put me in the tub. The contractions still felt like a tightening belt, but now it felt as if my muscles were getting sore from all the cramping, so things were hurting more.

"We call this an aquadural instead of an epidural," Doula explained. "The water is going to relax you, and the floating feeling will help with the pain."

I lay on my back in the tub, my giant belly floating. Under the tub was my hair clip, the one I hadn't been able to reach down and pick back up for a month because I was so pregnant. I could actually see my tummy tightening with the contractions, and I rubbed it as if to tell it everything was okay. Each contraction began to come with pressure, pain, breathing, and some weird sounds. I said things like, "Wow-wow-wow-wow," and "Yoooooooooooooooooo." I could tell Phillip was starting to get on edge, concerned that I was now so verbal with each contraction. His face looked confused and uncomfortable, as if he was no longer in control. Which, of course, he wasn't. He stayed near me, almost asking me with his face what he should do. As she had done all day, Doula asked me a series of questions: "Are you feeling the need to bear down?" she asked. "Is the pressure in your back coming and going with contractions? Can you feel the baby moving lower?"

"I don't know. I think so. I definitely feel the pressure moving down," I answered in between contractions. But I had no idea about anything else. Bear down? Like the Chicago Bears? I don't know.

Doula concluded that it was probably time to make our move. Her concern was that, if the contractions got much stronger, my water could break, and labor could progress very rapidly in the tub. And while I still admired home births, suddenly staring down the imminent passage of my son through my vagina removed the homebirth option from my short list for the day.

The ride to the hospital was pretty terrible. Phillip was driving like a bat out of hell, and in between contractions, I shouted from the back seat, "Don't get a ticket!" I'd seen those shows in which the husbands of women who were in labor got pulled over and they ended up delivering in the car.

At the hospital, I slowly walked, contracted, and walked again to Labor and Delivery. They checked us in and forced me to do a ridiculous number of things that no woman in labor should have to do. *Pee in a cup? Right now? This doesn't seem like the time. Lie flat on my back so that you can monitor my contractions? Lady, I can tell you myself when the contractions are coming. Just listen.*

The pain throughout these hospital intake rituals was horrible. I felt as if I was losing control. I looked at people walking past me—nurses and other hospital staff—wondering what they were thinking about me as I cried and held on to things. Tables, arms, walls—I grabbed anything I could use to hold me up as the pain welled up in my belly again and again. Doula helped me get onto the bed, and I curled up in the fetal position, breathing and staring at a green blinking light on a machine. I breathed and made an *ooooooh* sound each time I felt another contraction coming. Even through the pain, I was excited—thrilled even—that we were here, and it was time. I didn't feel the need to push. I just felt the need to breathe and try to regain control the way I had done during the first part of labor. I missed being able to regroup and prepare for the next contraction. They were coming too quickly now.

Then came the questions: "Who will be taking care of this baby when you get home? Do either of you use heroin? Does anyone in your family have cancer or acne?" Phillip answered everything as best he could while holding my hand and breathing with me. I began to get so aggravated with all the questioning that I started twisting and turning in the bed to get the contraction monitor to move so the nurse would have to reposition it and stop asking. Doula stayed at my head, reminding me to focus and breathe.

Finally, after an hour of questions and protocol, it was time to check my progress. I felt that I had to be at least eight centimeters, but I would settle for six. I pleaded with the nurse, "Gentle. Please be gentle," as I anticipated the pain of the next contraction. She checked. I waited. And finally … "Four and a half or so. That's good."

"*What?*" I screamed. "Four? I've been four since *Thursday!*"

"Oh, okay," she replied. "Well, let's see if you progress over the next hour, and then we'll formally admit you. If not, we can just send you home. It's best."

Send me home? Pardon my French, but are you fa-reaking kidding me? *I've been in labor for thirteen hours and you want to send me* home? I panicked, refused, and insisted I was having a baby.

But alas.

The massive letdown sent my body into hibernation. My contractions slowed to a stop.

We walked the hospital corridors and tried a few new positions, but nothing kicked me back into gear. My morale was completely obliterated. I went back to the room, collapsed onto the bed, and cried. The nurse checked me again. Fourteen hours and still four centimeters.

"This is normal for a first pregnancy," the nurse said kindly, but it didn't matter. I was sunk. And I was giving up. I felt like a complete and utter failure.

CHAPTER 31

The Labor I Needed

Does labor just stop?

Does this mean I need a C-section?

When will I know if they're going to induce me?

On top of feeling like a failure, I felt as if I knew nothing. By this time my mom and Phillip's entire family were at the hospital. My birthing plan was already out the window, and I couldn't see how anything after this would be close to what I had envisioned for myself. I was embarrassed that everyone had come and I didn't have anything to show them. I always said I'd be fine with whatever way Abraham decided to make his entrance into the world. But I'd said that with one caveat: I needed to *know* how he would do it. I was left with the ultimate answer: I know nothing. I control nothing.

Before I left the hospital that Saturday night, the nurses all suggested I take something to help me relax and sleep for the night, as I would need my strength for the next day if labor were to continue. Doula agreed it might be a good idea. I rolled over and took one of the most painful shots in my behind I'd *ever* felt. (How was *that* supposed to relax me?) This shot was a muscle relaxer, and while my body chilled out, the nurses put me in a wheelchair and pushed me to the exit. My in-laws all walked with me and told me not to worry, that it was all normal, and everything would be fine. I smiled and tried to believe them.

Defeated.

It was midnight. I lay on my bed with Doula, and my contractions started again, this time very far apart and not as intense. Doula suggested we call my chiropractor (the hippy dippy one) to see if she would make a house call to help me loosen my pelvic muscles and help me relax some more. Amazingly, she raced to our house with her suitcase of tools in the middle of the night.

The muscle relaxer didn't kill the contractions, but it did make me high as a kite. I flowed in and out of crying and sleeping and breathing through contractions, which were now about every ten minutes again. My chiropractor worked on me for forty minutes, none of which I clearly remember except for the moment her head disconnected from her body and floated over my face repeating, "You're doing great!"

Was it the best choice to have accepted the muscle relaxer? I still can't say for certain. It did help me relax, though I still felt every contraction and only slept in ten-minute intervals over the next four hours. Looking back, I can say for certain that the muscle relaxer didn't interfere or have any side effects, so maybe it was a good choice. It did enable me to just zone out for a while.

Doula left around midnight, along with the chiropractor. Phillip fell asleep. I was alone, next to Phillip, falling asleep and then waking up to a contraction and falling back asleep every ten minutes.

At about three in the morning, the contractions picked up some speed and strength. I began working hard to breathe through them again. I hadn't eaten since lunch the day before (*The Hangover* now seemed like a months-old memory) and had barely drunk anything since leaving for the hospital. Phillip woke up when he heard my heavy breathing. I was still lying on my side (trying to sleep, which was adorable). I'm not sure how Phillip felt in this moment, but knowing that Doula wasn't there to coach *him*, he knew he had to coach me.

"Breathe. Breath. Good. You sound great," he whispered. "Do you want to try sitting on the toilet again?"

I felt extremely irritable. The pain was pain, and I could almost deal with that. I was having trouble with the waves of unknown that swept over me with each contraction. My stomach would tense, the pain would set in, I would panic not knowing if this was the contraction that would break my water, and then after about a minute the pain would soften, and I would breathe.

"I guess so," I responded in between contractions and slowly got up to sit on the toilet.

He texted Doula, and she suggested that he run a bath again. Phillip gently eased me into the warm water, and I started to cry. The pain increased. Fast. It was like nothing I'd ever felt. I floated there, writhing with each contraction. I looked Phillip in the eye and apologized because I couldn't do it anymore. "I tried," I told him over and over again.

Of course, it didn't make any sense, so he didn't know how to respond. It wasn't like trying to tie a square knot and failing so the captain of the sailboat just does it for you. There was no one else who could do this for me. But I think in that moment, I wanted to believe someone else could do the rest for me, so I kept apologizing for failing and telling him I had tried. I was just waiting for someone to hug me and tell me it was over.

Phillip got me out of the tub at around four thirty. At this point, I was angry. I began pacing the house. My mom heard me and came out of the guest room, but she didn't come near me or talk to me. I entered a primal state of being, grunting and groaning, and ignoring everyone and everything around me.

I felt really angry that no one was making this easier. No one was tying the square knot for me. Phillip tried standing in front of me with food and water. At one point he even offered me a sandwich. I shouted, "I hate crust!" and pushed past him. I've never had a problem with sandwich crusts, not even as a kid, but at the moment it was the only control I had.

And I knew that Phillip and my mother felt even more helpless than I did, but when you are in such an enormous life transition, your codependency goes away. It was like running a marathon and being so thirsty that you just get tunnel vision; you just keep moving your blistered feet forward until you find water, because it's literally life and death. I couldn't see outside a very small field, and I didn't need to. Even the deepest meditations, the quietest spaces, the most reflective moments—nothing before or since compared to that completely overwhelming primal state in which I could do nothing but keep breathing. That was a wonderful lesson—which I recognized only afterwards, of course—that everybody survived when I wasn't taking care of them.

Doula came back at about five thirty in the morning, shortly after I threw myself on the bed in the middle of a contraction. I could hear her and Phillip whispering over me while I rolled and twisted in agony, but I never caught anything they said. I remember thinking that I hoped they were both in agreement that labor was over and I could go eat some chicken noodle soup. I even sat up after a contraction and announced I was finished and I was going to the table to eat a meal.

The trouble with labor is that, no matter how hard you try, you can't stop it. The end to the pain comes when it wants to, not when you decide.

I labored through the worst four hours of my life there in my bedroom. I cried and screamed and begged Doula to make it stop. She continued changing my positions and suggesting new alternatives.

In the end, I found myself in the tub again. I screamed in desperation, "*Take me to the hospital!*" Doula asked me what was going to happen at the hospital, and I snapped that I didn't know, I just needed to go somewhere. I needed to do something different. Doula looked me in the eye as the sunlight beginning to peek through the bathroom window and said, "If you do three contractions in the squatting position, we'll go to the hospital."

I looked straight back and asked, "Are you fucking kidding me?"

She shook her head. "I want your water to break," she whispered. "I want your labor to progress. Now let's do three contractions. You're doing great."

I did those three contractions in the squatting position and, like a lioness, roared through the house to the car. I don't remember the second ride to the hospital. Neither do I remember the security guard who apparently told Phillip to just park in an ambulance parking spot in front because he was so fearful of the noises I was making. Phillip said he thought I was dying. I do remember being pushed in a wheelchair straight to Labor and Delivery and walking directly to the same room I'd left. I didn't even stop to ask where to go. That was my room, and I was taking it back.

It was nine in the morning on Sunday. I'd been in labor for twenty-five hours.

Of course, I was immediately given instructions to pee in a cup and put on a gown and get hooked up to the monitors. There was absolutely no way I could do any of these things, and when I went completely mental on the nurse who tried to help me into the bathroom (I think I shouted, "You know I can't even pee!"), she backed up as if I was the star of *The Exorcist*. "Okay, no problem, sweetie. You don't have to pee in the cup. It's fine."

I made it back to the bed and felt the worst contraction yet. It hurt to cry, and it hurt to breathe, and Doula grabbed me under my arms and let me hang beneath her, my body limp on the floor. It was truly one of the most humiliating moments of the entire experience; hanging there like a rag doll, no control, sobbing and screaming while the nurses and Phillip stared. As soon as one contraction finished and I thought I had caught my breath, another came.

I screamed through two-minute-long, body-rocking contractions. Phillip and Doula lifted me to the bed. I couldn't think while I searched for any surface, anything that might brace me and make the pain more manageable before the next one came. I knew people were around me— holding me even—but I didn't know who was where; neither did I care. Everything became disoriented, and it didn't matter who was doing what. When a contraction ended, I would look at the nearest person, begging her or him with my eyes to tell me that I was okay, that this pain was normal. And then, another one would come.

Nurses began furiously poking me with needles in my left arm. I wasn't sure why this was happening now as opposed to last night until I heard one nurse comment that I was spilling ketones in my urine and was extremely dehydrated. I didn't remember peeing, so I wasn't sure how she knew this, but as the next contraction came, I didn't care. My body sucked down a liter of saline in eight minutes (according to Phillip). They put up another bag immediately and another one after that. The nurse, a middle-aged woman with kind eyes, too much mascara, and a sweet southern voice, laid her head next to mine on the bed even though she was standing up. "Erin?" she said. "Sweetie, I read your birth plan. We can easily accommodate everything for you, but I want you to know right now that pain medication is available to you if you need a break. I won't ask you about it again after this."

Doula told the nurse I'd been in labor since eight in the morning the day before, and she felt that it may be time for me to accept some help. "She'd probably benefit from an epidural to get through delivery," Doula said softly after I screamed through another contraction.

"I think so too," the nurse gently agreed. "We can certainly do that for her. Mama deserves a break."

This had not been the plan. The plan had been for me to be a superhero and finish the job myself. This was what women were made to do, and I was going to do it and carry the bragging rights in my pocket forever. I couldn't surrender. It wouldn't be my perfect birth. I said all of that to Doula with my eyes and she stared hard right back at me. Hard. Then she said the words that completely changed my life. "Erin, you get the labor you need. You don't have to be perfect. You're allowed to take the help."

I cried through the next contraction, feeling half like a loser and half like a woman finally free of a lifetime striving to make all the equations fit. It all hit me at once like a huge emotional release I'd been carrying my entire life. It was finally time for me to admit that being a hero didn't mean writing all the equations myself.

I continued to cry in pain and a little in relief through the following contractions while the nurse checked my progress. Twenty-six hours in, I was eight centimeters. My cervix was 100 percent thinned out, or as they called it in labor and delivery, effaced. Abe was near the bottom of my cervix.

The nurse smiled and got close to my face again. "Do you know how well you've done? It's time for you to rest so that you can push this baby out."

I nodded and accepted help genuinely and from my heart with no ego. I'd been broken. There was no energy for ego.

Stripped down to my soul, I felt a peace I'd never felt. I wasn't disappointed that I hadn't achieved the goals I had written down on paper. In fact, my feelings were quite the opposite. I was proud. In that moment, I began to see the beauty, strength, and courage in myself that I'd only pretended to see before. I couldn't become a mom without accepting help. That was my lesson. That was the labor I needed.

The anesthesiologist arrived within seconds, it seemed. He was a small, thin man with professional glasses. He carefully explained to me everything he would be doing, but I really don't remember any of the words.

I saw Phillip sitting on a bench in front of me with Doula during another contraction. Phillip was crying, scared for me. He later told me that was the worst moment of the entire experience. He said my eyes didn't just communicate pain—they screamed with fear. And he was right. I was terrified. I didn't know it, but he had to leave the room at one point to keep from losing it while I got the epidural.

The kind nurse held me as I sat on the edge of the bed through contractions. It took the anesthesiologist five tries to get the epidural into my spine. Five pokes, five contractions, almost seven long minutes. The nurse kept pushing my head down into my stomach so that my spine would stretch and separate. I am such a small person that it took an act of God to spread my vertebrae enough to get the needle in. The anesthesiologist tried to administer a local anesthetic so that I would not feel the needle going in, but after I screamed, "*I can feel everything!*" and realized that I was only slowing him down, I decided that feeling a needle going into my spine was the trade-off for ultimate relief.

I kid you not—within minutes, the epidural took effect. I closed my eyes, tears streaming down my face, and breathed as fully and calmly as I could. It had been almost twenty-six hours since I'd been able do that. Doula rubbed my forehead before deciding it was a nice time for Phillip and me to be alone. But before I could really even acknowledge him in the room, I dozed off.

The nap was short, maybe about twenty minutes. But when the nurse woke me up to check me again, I felt a new mental preparedness for what would come next.

I should let you know that when I say "the nurse" I am talking about one of at least four of them. I cannot, to this day, remember any of them except for the kind nurse with a lot of mascara who told me it was okay to accept help. One thing about labor and delivery—there are a lot of people who come in and out of your room in the hospital, and very few of them introduce themselves.

The nurse smiled. "Ten centimeters! You're ready to start pushing. Do you want to try to push now?"

I was so shocked and excited that Abe was ready! After such a long trial getting to this point, it seemed quick now! I tried to push but couldn't feel anything. "Am I pushing?"

The nurse sweetly replied. "Not really."

I focused hard on my body and the muscles I needed to use to push Abe out. I tried again and again until on the fourth time, the nurse said, "Oh! That's it! That was a push!"

Pushing basically felt like I was half trying to poop and half trying to pee. It wasn't really a feeling I'd experienced before, and no one tells you that pushing isn't always a natural feeling when you first start.

Annie had agreed to be on call for me through the weekend despite the fact that she wasn't working. She'd arrived at the hospital shortly after I did, for which I was so thankful. The last thing I wanted was Old Man Winter there with his C-Section shirt on.

The nurses quickly dismantled the bed and set up trays of metal instruments and plastic bins. Doula entered the room and took a seat off to the side. During this time, Phillip and I took a moment to reflect and even cry about how amazing and exciting this was. I was so grateful to be engaged and alert enough to be present in that moment. It is my favorite memory of Abe's birth.

"He's coming!" Phillip said to me.

"I know. Finally!"

"Can you feel that contraction?" Phillip asked, looking at the monitor.

"No! I can't feel my stomach at all."

"That's amazing!"

The nurse continued to instruct me to push with each contraction. I couldn't feel the contractions, but I could definitely feel the pain of Abe's head descending down the canal. My pushing got better and better as I figured out which muscles to use. "Oh, she's a good little pusher!" one nurse said. "Time to get down to business!"

Doula held one leg, I held the other, and Phillip sat behind me supporting my head. I had asked for a mirror in my birth plan, which turned out to be extremely helpful. I could see what was working and what wasn't with each push. Phillip could also see everything that was happening without leaving my head. (A lot of people are completely freaked out by the mirror, so I just include this detail to tell you that it was an awesome motivator.)

I moved Abe down the canal so quickly that the nurse told me to stop and wait for a moment.

When my midwife took her position between my legs with a flashlight on her head and really long gloves, Old Man Winter came waltzing through the door. He just happened to be in the neighborhood on a Sunday and thought he would stop by. I figure that, convinced I would be having a C-section, he asked to be informed when I was admitted so that he could perform it. I'm not sure I spoke to him or even acknowledged him for the brief moment he was there. I just pushed as hard and as long as I could to show him I didn't need him.

Eventually I remember him putting his hand on my shoulder and smiling. "You're doing great." That felt awesome.

Pushing got more painful each time, and I began to let out those primitive grunts you hear women making on TV. The pressure and pain in my pelvis was incredible. It hurt so much, almost like a really big poop. You know you will feel *so* good once it's out … except it was taking a really long time to get it out. Sometimes the midwife would count three pushes, and I would throw in an extra fourth before the contraction was over. I began to repeat from my gut, "Get him out. I have to get him out." The epidural definitely numbed my tummy, but I could still feel everything from the waist down.

And then, the room went blurry.

I could still hear voices, but no longer was I a part of it all. I entered a canal of my own, staring into the mirror and watching my baby come close to the edge and then disappear again. I could see nothing but my canal, the mirror, and my baby's head as I pushed.

"Erin! Reach down and feel his head! He has so much hair!" someone murmured in the distance. I reached down because I was told to, but I didn't really put effort into feeling. I just kept pushing.

"You're almost there! He's turning the corner!"

A huge and tremendous rush of pain overtook me as I felt Abraham's head coming through my pelvis. This was the hardest part, as it was not a fluid movement. He would move forward, and then back just a little bit. And I could somehow feel all of it. In a moment of screaming and pushing, the pain got so bad that I closed my eyes and I thought to myself, "This has *got* to be his head coming out."

I went inside myself to push with everything I had. I don't remember anyone telling me the head was out, or that his shoulder was out, or that he was born. I don't remember Doula shouting, "Grab your baby!" I remember pushing until I looked down on my stomach and there he was. There was the person I'd been waiting to meet, pink as a rose and loud as a train.

"You did it!" I cried to Abe as I looked at him in disbelief.

Phillip cut the cord and followed Abe to the scale with a nurse, and then to the warmer where the nurses tended to him for five long minutes. Doula was at my side, smiling. I remember her saying, "Isn't this cool, Erin?" while I breathed and laughed and cried and reached for my baby. Phillip smiled and giggled and laughed, following Abe around the nurses with his camera. I still felt half-primal, half in a weird bubble where everything looked blurry and I just wanted my baby in my arms, all while feeling so, so happy.

Finally, the nurse handed Abe to me, and I placed him on my chest. I breathed. He didn't cry. Here he was. I closed my eyes. Everything was quiet. And everything felt finished and also as if life had just started. I thought of nothing. I longed for nothing.

My baby is here.

Life was never life until he fit right there beneath my chin.

Epilogue — 2018

Whether you've been told you have PCOS, endometriosis, unexplained infertility, or if you've experienced multiple heart-breaking miscarriages, there is no relief until you hold a baby in your arms. Until then, *infertility* is a dirty word. It's not a topic you can bring up at cocktail parties, it's uncomfortable to discuss with your family, it's impossible to explain to your boss ("I'll be out three days this week for internal ultrasounds."), and it's an almost unbearable thing to tell your friends who have kids. And the cruel, cruel trick is that just the word *infertility* makes your entire body yearn for a child more than you ever thought possible. I know this to be true.

If you're a woman struggling with any form of infertility, I want to tell you that it will not turn out the way you always hoped. It will be harder, funnier, weirder, longer, more stressful, more interesting, and far less in your control than any story you could tell yourself about having a baby. But when you do hold that baby in your arms, whether he or she is from your body or from someone else's, you will not remember the struggle the way you fear you will. You won't be defined by it; neither will your little one. And if, after trying for long enough, you no longer want to try, it doesn't mean you gave up. It doesn't mean you failed. You aren't less of a woman because having a baby *wasn't* more important than your mental or physical health. You are strong and amazing and the owner of your life story. Many women aren't, so savor that decision and feel proud of it. And maybe be an awesome auntie someday.

As I finish writing this book, Abraham is now seven. In the morning, he still likes to find ways to fit beneath my chin, only now he is standing when he does it. Like trying to conceive a child, or enduring a high-risk pregnancy and a labor with a mind of its own, life and marriage take you

215

places you'd never expect. I think it's important to tell you but not harp on the fact that Phillip and I are no longer married. There is no juicy story; neither is there a scandal. In that way, writing this book was a cathartic confirmation that we made the right choice. Though it still makes me really sad.

We live just a few miles apart now, each very happily remarried, sharing our son with as much kindness and honesty as possible.

Abraham, though … he is the sun and the moon and the stars. He loves storytelling, drawing, electronics, puppies, and laughing his head off. He is a joyful human being. And I can tell you, with everything in me that's true, that I have never once looked at him and thought about the way he came into the world. He was so clearly and purposefully meant for me that my struggle to bring him here was only a lesson, not a punishment or a less-than-legitimate beginning. And Abe was kind enough to wait for me to learn that lesson before he made his entrance.

Being a mom has been a constant reminder that I am not in control. My job is not to control my son, only to guide him and show him how to live life by the way I live mine. This is not to say there are no rules in our house. Having no rules would only teach him that he is in control, and the last thing I want is for him to think that and then be supremely disappointed the first time life doesn't comply.

I am now a wife, a mom, and a *step*-mom. Blended families are no joke. This part of my life has stripped back more of the life equation I had for myself. I'm actually learning now that when I completely surrender to what's happening, opting only to move on what feels "good" instead of what feels "right," life can taste better than any meal I ever dreamed of cooking. It's more of a close-your-eyes-and-open-your-mouth kind of meal now. The surprises are always sweet. But that's another book for another time.

I, myself, chose not to have more children. It's a decision I simultaneously praise God for and also deeply regret. While I have no idea whether or not my body would be willing to play along here in my second marriage, it was a joint decision that adding another one to our crew wouldn't fit the family and life we've built. But I will always wonder if I could have gotten pregnant naturally as so many women do after their first pregnancy is an effort. Just because you have one child doesn't mean the wondering ever stops.

Abraham's debut was equally about giving birth to myself as it was giving birth to him. I have been reborn again and again in the days and years since he joined me, sometimes finding amazing parts of me coming to life, and sometimes releasing huge parts that I never thought would go away. He is my heart, made from my blood, raised in my love. My prayer is that, while he remains a constant in my life, he will continue to grow away from me. As heartbreaking as it is, this story about my sacrifice to conceive and give birth to him comes on the heels of knowing the only goal thereafter is to lovingly help him leave me one day. It's crazy that any of us even want to do this thing called motherhood.

But we do, don't we?

We want it more than life itself sometimes.